Children's Understandings of Well-Being

Saoirse Nic Gabhainn
Jane Sixsmith
June 2005

On behalf of the research team and administrative support:
Simon Comer, Ailish Houlihan, Siobhan O'Higgins, Tommy Gannon,
Colette Fleming, Mary Cooke, Christina Costello and Efah Samuel

Centre for Health Promotion Studies
Department of Health Promotion
National University of Ireland, Galway

The National Children's Office,
1st Floor, St. Martin's House, Waterloo Road, Dublin 4
Tel: 353 1 242 0000 Fax: 353 1 664 1929
Email: nco@health.gov.ie Website: www.nco.ie

Design: Penhouse Design www.penhouse.ie
Printed by: New Oceans

01

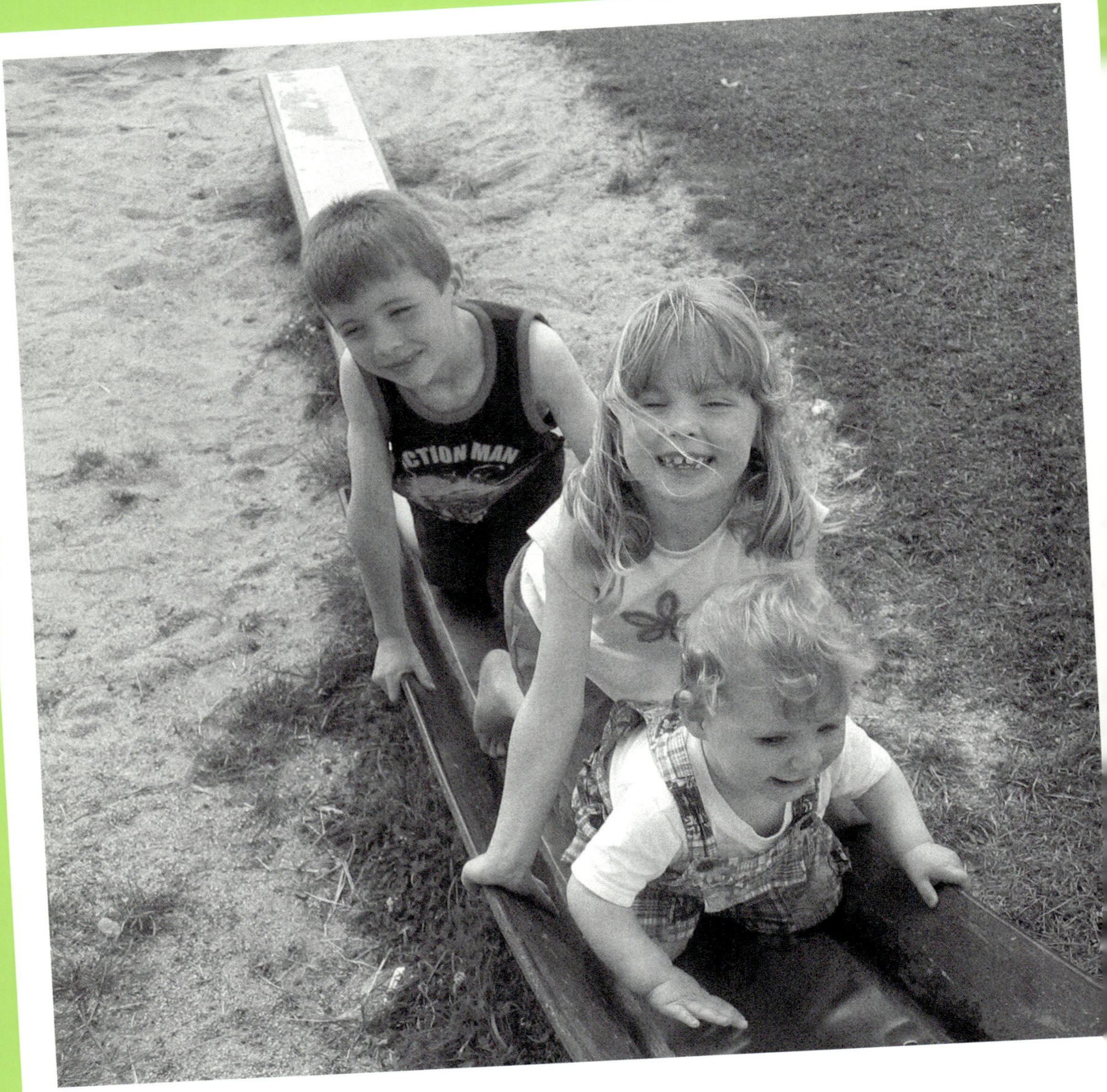

CONTENTS

03

LIST OF TABLES

LIST OF FIGURES

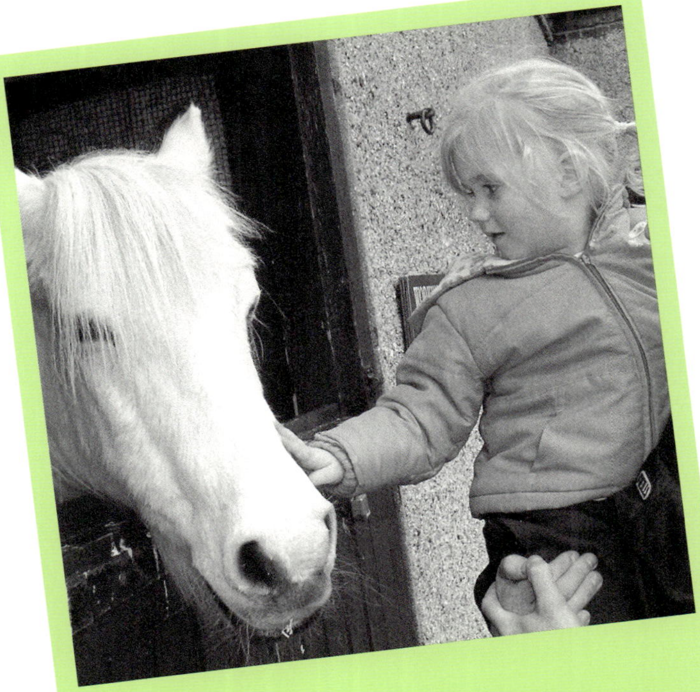

05

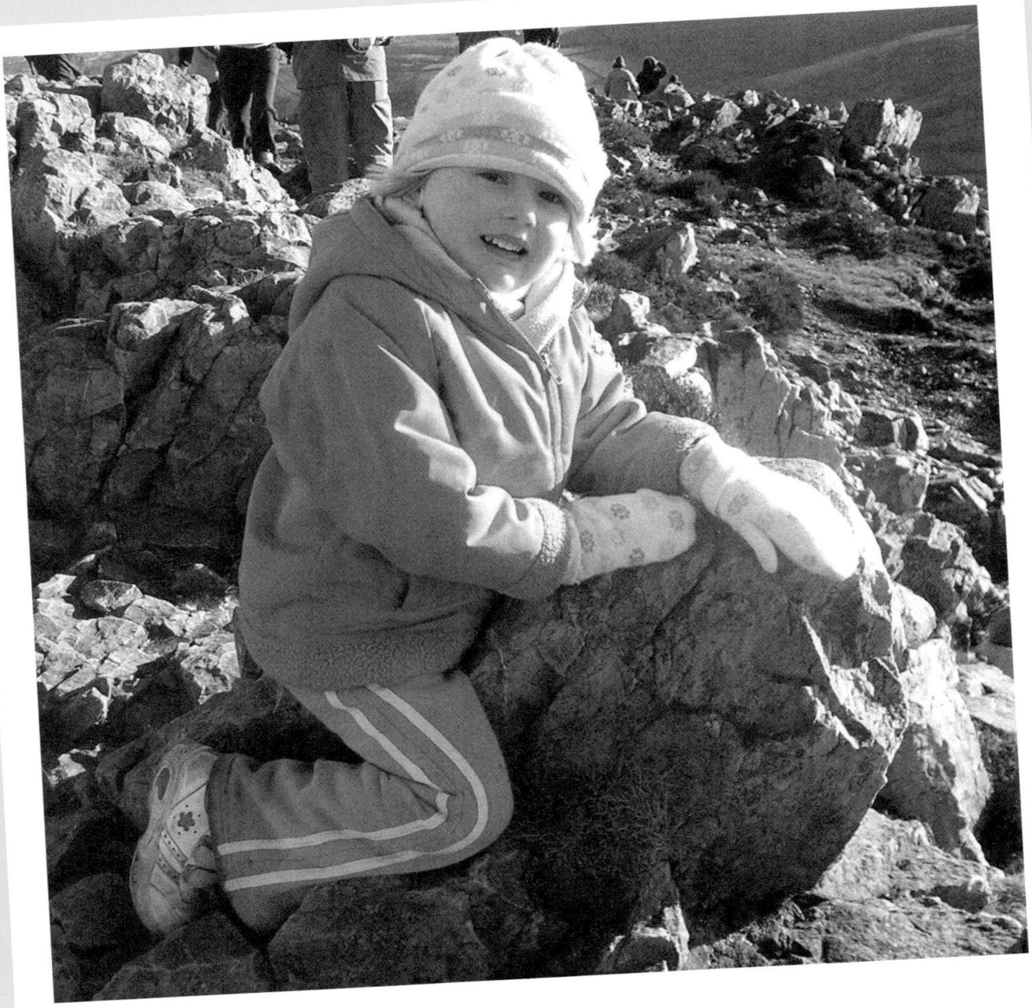

INTRODUCTION

A global commitment to improve child well-being was included in the 1989 UN Convention on the Rights of the Child (United Nations, 1989) and the deployment of appropriate indicators at a country or regional level has been recognised as a vital step towards this goal.

In Ireland the National Children's Strategy (2000) outlines three key goals:

1. CHILDREN WILL HAVE A VOICE;
2. CHILDREN'S LIVES WILL BE BETTER UNDERSTOOD;
3. CHILDREN WILL RECEIVE QUALITY SUPPORTS AND SERVICES.

The development of National Child Well-Being Indicators has been set out as a key action under the National Children's Strategy (2000). This research aims to contribute to the development of National Child Well-Being Indicators. It is a sister piece of research to a Delphi Study being conducted by research staff within the National Children's Office to achieve consensus on well-being indicators. The National Children's Office agreed that it would not be appropriate to include children in the Delphi study and thus they called for tenders for a study on children's understandings of well-being. It was specifically suggested that a group approach to data collection and analysis be taken (NCO, 2003). The approach chosen and developed is explicitly intended to be coherent with the overall goals of the National Children's Strategy. The research described in this report is designed to give children a voice in the development of well-being indicators and in doing so, to provide data that will help children's lives be better understood.

This report contains a short contextual introduction, which is followed by details of the methods employed during the research. The procedural information is integrated with the findings. It moves sequentially through the main phases of the research, from design and sampling issues, through the photography phase to the schema development phase. Finally, conclusions are drawn.

CONTEXT

Well-being, according to several authors (e.g. Diener, 1984; Huebner, 1991; Wilkinson and Walford, 1998), is multi-faceted. Absence of distress is a major component, but equally important is the presence of positive affective states, such as happiness. An important aspect of well-being is one's overall evaluation of life, or life satisfaction. Thus in quantitative surveys of well-being, measures of self-rated health, self-reported happiness, global life satisfaction and the presence of distress, or symptoms, are frequently included (e.g. Torsheim et al., 2001).

The World Health Organisation defines physical, mental and social well-being as major components of health (WHO, 1946). Thus health is not merely the absence of disease, but the presence of positive health. As Bowling (1995, p. 7) points out, the concept of positive health implies 'completeness', 'full-functioning' or mental and physical 'efficiency', as well as social competence and adjustment, but beyond this there is no accepted definition (Tones and Tilford, 2001). Neither is there agreement on whether health should be conceptualised as unidimenional, with positive health at one end and negative health at the other, or whether there are independent dimensions (Downie et al., 1990; Diener, 1984). Independent or not, they have been found to be highly correlated in adolescent populations (Wilkinson and Walford, 1998).

O'Higgins (2002) interviewed 31 first-year post-primary school pupils about their perceptions of happiness and health. She reports that among these Irish children, both happiness and health are perceived to be associated with physical participation in life, while unhappiness is associated with difficulties in relationships with others. Being strong enough, able-bodied enough or having sufficient energy to pursue plans for participating in life were the key issues that the young people identified as being related to health. Happiness was associated to a greater extent with spending time with friends and taking part in life. A sense of belonging within families and communities also emerged as important aspects of happiness. Gender differences were identified, with girls reporting more involvement with, and greater impact on their health and happiness from interpersonal relationships than did boys, while boys were more likely than girls to report the importance of their future plans and sense of anticipation of life events to come. Both boys and girls recognised that their current preoccupations and concerns may not be stable and were likely to change over time.

Irish children, surveyed as part of the 2002 Health Behaviour in School-aged Children Survey (Kelleher et al., 2003), report relatively high levels of self-rated health and happiness. Of the 10-17 year olds surveyed, 86% reported that their health is good or excellent, while 88% report that they are very or quite happy with their lives. These overall figures mask some important gender and age differences. Girls are less likely to report being very happy than boys and are also less likely to report that their health is excellent. In addition, self-reported health and happiness decreases notably with age amongst the girls and decreases less so amongst boys. No consistent differences are found across social class groups. Glynn (2002) identified that among Irish school children, psychological and emotional factors were more predictive of subjective well-being and life satisfaction than were physical factors. He identified an indicator of subjective health, 'feeling low', as most predictive, in a negative sense, of well-being, happiness and life satisfaction.

The research in this report builds on these investigations which have taken place in the Centre for Health Promotion Studies, NUI Galway. We have employed a population-based survey to look at socio-demographic differences in self-rated health, happiness and life satisfaction among children and adolescents, identifying differences between genders and age groups (Kelleher et al., 2003). We have also identified that, among Irish youth, psychological and social health appears to be more predictive of these measures of well-being than does physical health, absence of distress or involvement in health-promoting behaviours (Glynn, 2002). Gender differences also emerged in O'Higgins' (2002) qualitative approach to this subject, but involvement in life and relationships with others were most important in her participants' perspectives of well-being. This study aims to be gender-balanced and to include boys and girls separately and together, as well as to build other socio-demographic characteristics, namely age and urban/rural location, into the research design.

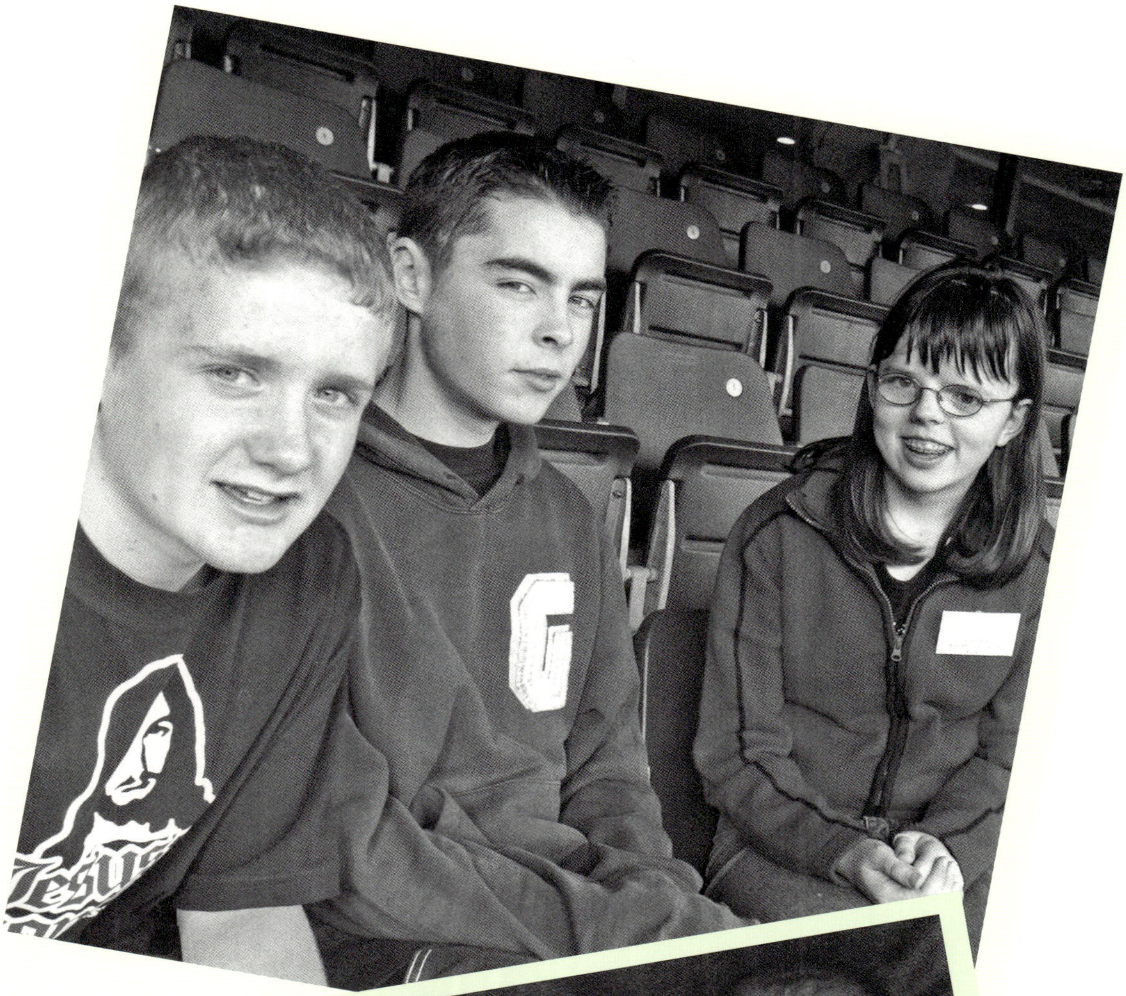

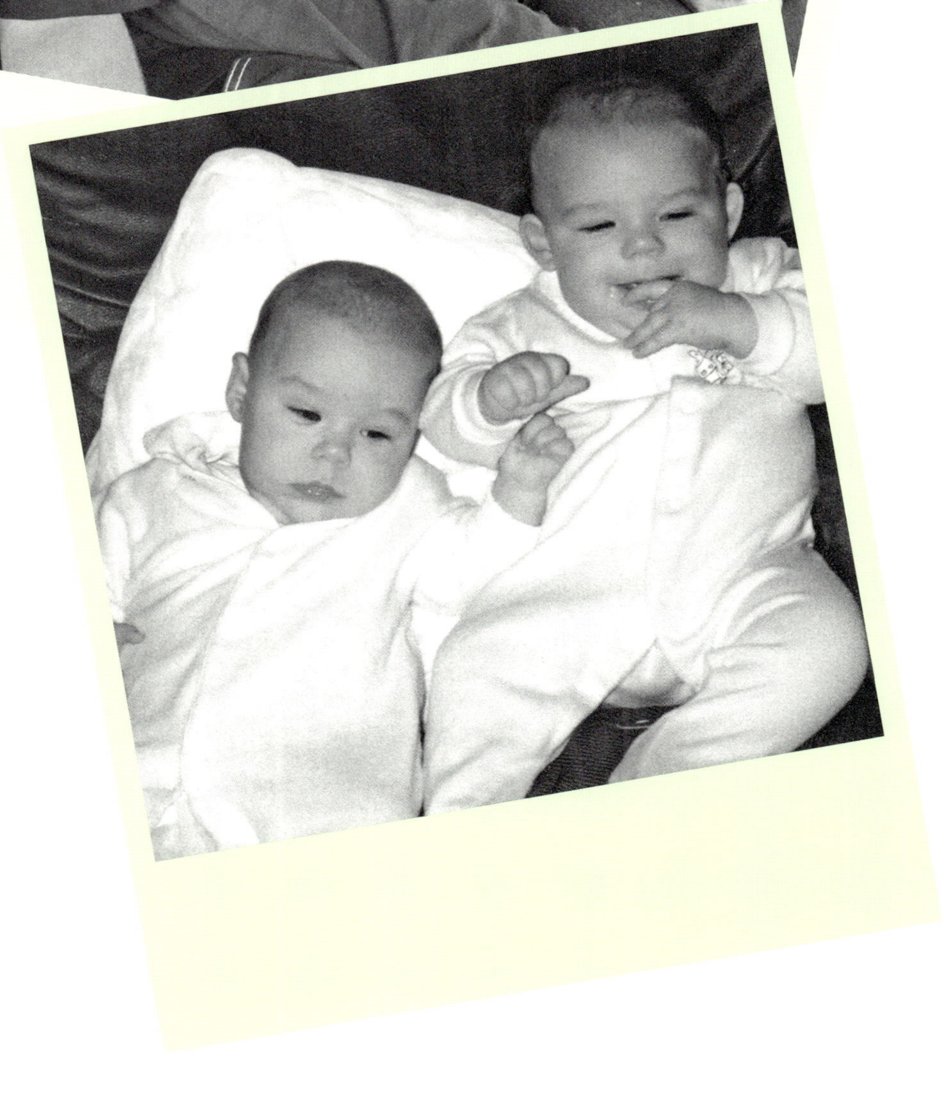

08

09

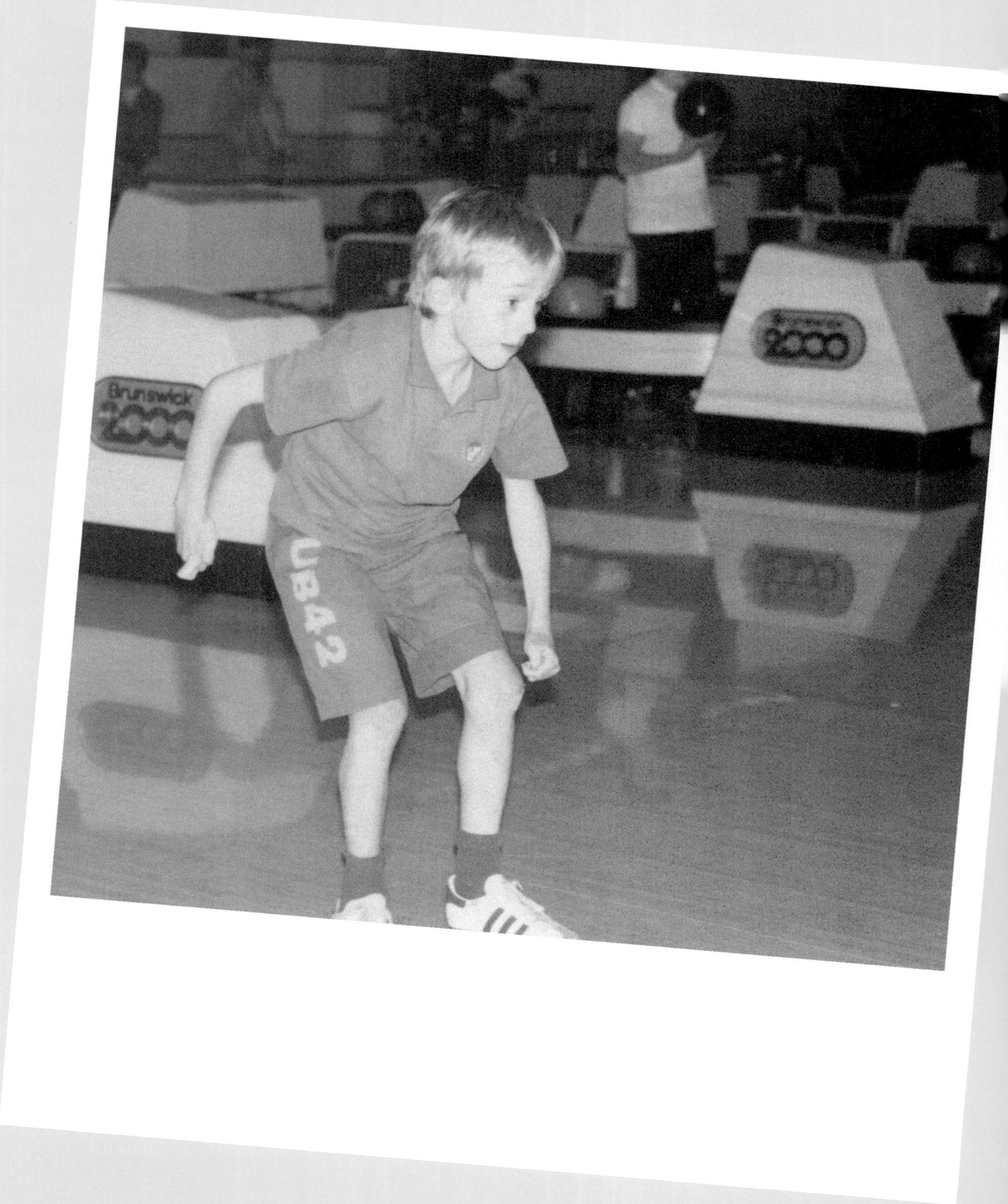

METHODS

This section introduces the procedures, study design and the sampling procedures adopted. There are three main components to the study. The first involves the use of disposable cameras by children. Class groups of children were shown how to use a disposable camera and asked to take photographs of things, people or places that *"make them well"* or *"keep them well".* The cameras provided took up to 27 colour photographs. Once developed, the photographs were returned to the children who had taken them and they were asked to annotate them. A full set of their own photographs and the single set of negatives were returned to each child. The second component involves groups of children looking at the developed photographs and dividing them into groups of mutually exclusive categories. The third component involves further groups of children in developing schematic representations, or schemata, of well-being, using photographic examples of the categories. These schemata are first developed by single gender groups, then by mixed gender groups. A final integration by a group of older young people is designed to provide a comprehensive representation of well-being relevant to Irish children.

The process adopted was initially piloted among primary school children in urban and rural settings. The main objectives were to assess the feasibility of the proposed procedures, particularly during the classroom and group sessions. The pilot study illustrated the feasibility of the camera demonstration in the classroom, the required processing time for the cameras and developed photographs, the class time and level of assistance required to facilitate the annotation of photographs and the feasibility of the categorisation and schema development phases even with primary school children. Following the pilot study a number of changes were made: an initial proposal to brainstorm the meaning of well-being with children was replaced by a period of quiet reflection; children were provided with self-adhesive labels for the cameras in order to label them by name, gender and age; and the instructions for annotating the developed photographs were refined.

DESIGN

The design of this study incorporates individual level data collection, three sets of group level data analysis and feedback with a final group level integration process.

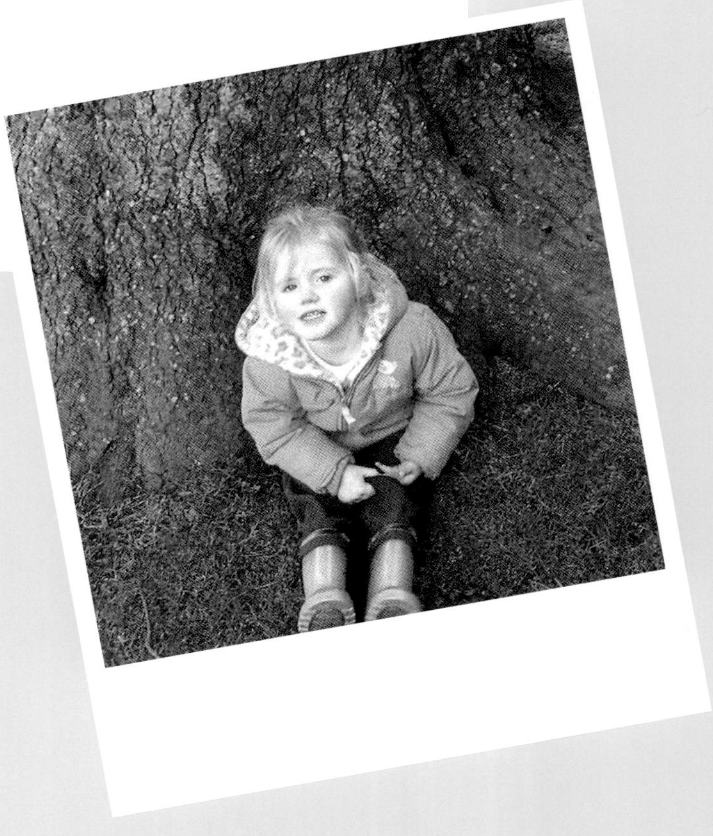

TABLE 1: Study design

FINAL INTEGRATION	FINAL INTEGRATION: YOUTH CENTRE (SENIOR CYCLE ONLY)															
Schema development	Urban 5th class [Boys, Girls, Mixed]				Rural 5th class [Boys, Girls, Mixed]				Urban TY [Boys, Girls, Mixed]				Rural TY [Boys, Girls, Mixed]			
Categorising	Urban 5th class boys		Urban 5th class girls		Rural 5th class boys		Rural 5th class girls		Urban TY boys		Urban TY girls		Rural TY boys		Rural TY girls	
Photographs	Urban 3rd class boys	Urban 5th class boys	Urban 3rd class girls	Urban 5th class girls	Rural 3rd class boys	Rural 5th class boys	Rural 3rd class girls	Rural 5th class girls	Urban 2nd year boys	Urban TY boys	Urban 2nd year girls	Urban TY girls	Rural 2nd year boys	Rural TY boys	Rural 2nd year girls	Rural TY girls

This design should be read from the bottom line up. The first line represents the individual classroom visited and the groups of children who took photographs as part of this study. The next line up represents the gender-specific groups of children who were involved in categorising the photographs taken. The next line (second from the top) represents the groups who were involved in the development of schemata and the top line represents the group of youth centre committee members who were involved in the final integration of the various models and schemata developed by other children and young people.

SAMPLE

For the first three phases of this research, children were accessed through schools. School lists were downloaded from the Department of Education and Science website. Separate lists were employed for Galway primary schools, Galway post-primary schools, Dublin primary schools and Dublin post-primary schools. Schools were randomly selected using a table of random numbers. Dublin schools were randomly selected from those identified as being located in Dublin City rather than in Fingal, Dun Laoghaire-Rathdown or Dublin South. The rationale was to ensure that the schools were located in and primarily drew their pupils from urban settings. Galway schools were randomly selected from schools within Galway County Borough. All Galway schools were outside the Galway City boundaries but within a 20-mile radius of Galway City. In this case the rationale was to ensure a primarily rural population base.

Within each geographical area and school type (primary/post-primary), those schools selected first were allocated to the initial photographs stage (phase 1). If a single sex school was selected, a second school of the same type but with pupils of the other sex was selected. The next set of schools selected was allocated to the categorisation stage (phase 2) and the last selected schools were allocated to the schema development stage (phase 3). All schools in phases 2 and 3 were required to be co-educational. A number of extra schools were selected in order to obviate the need to return to the sampling frame should any school be unwilling to participate, thus sampling with replacement was undertaken.

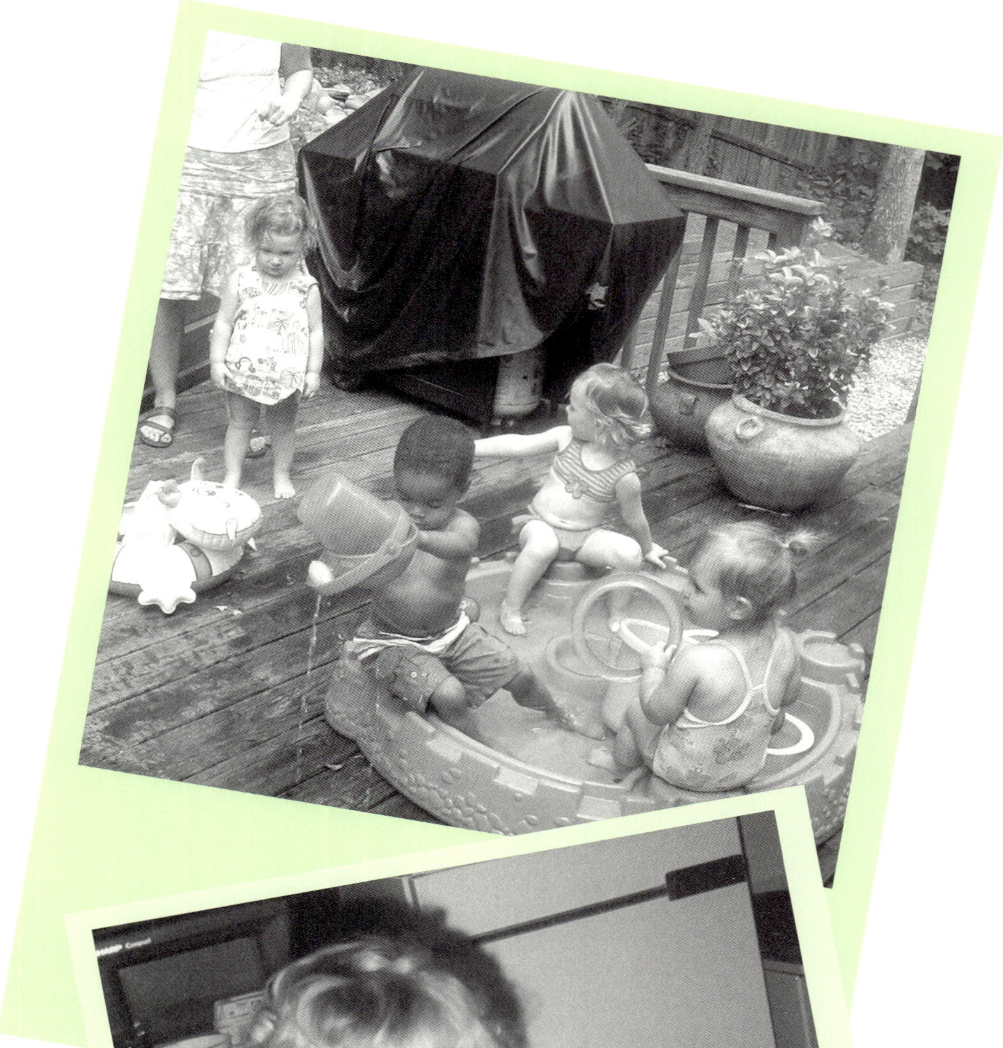

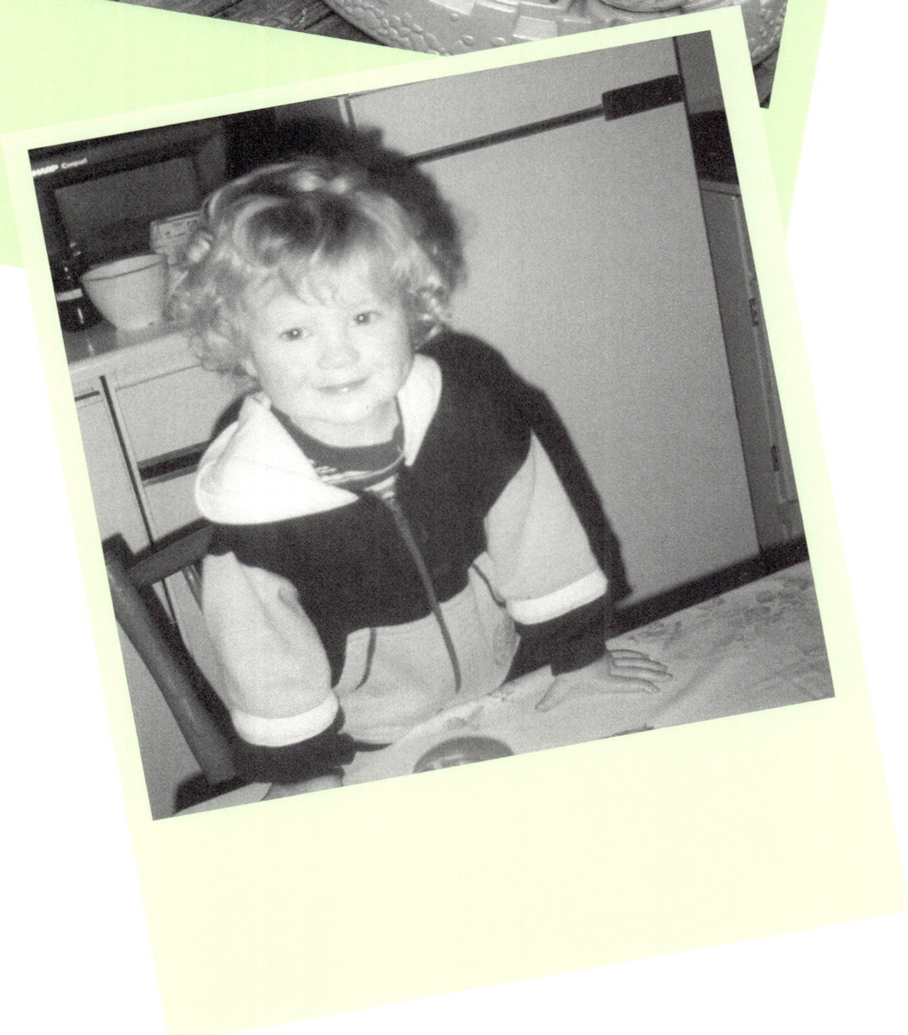

12

13

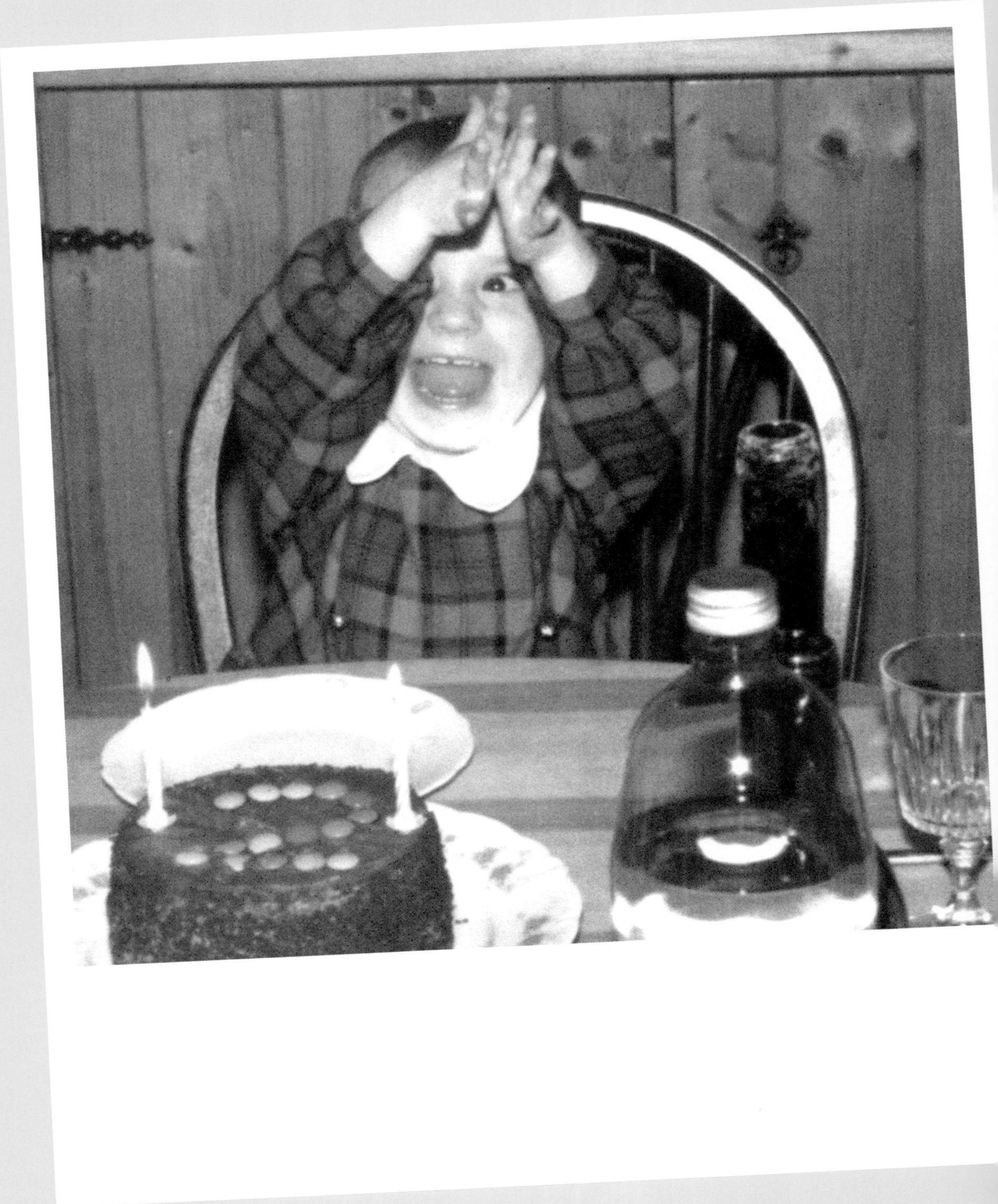

PROCEDURES AND RESULTS

The school principal in each of the selected schools was originally written to and invited to participate in this research exercise. Each principal was provided with a document outlining the rationale and procedures involved. Primary schools were asked to facilitate the participation of both 3rd and 5th class and post-primary schools 2nd year and the first year post-junior certificate. One principal immediately declined the invitation. Letters were followed up with a phone call and principals were asked to nominate a contact staff member from within the school. In almost all cases, the contact was the teacher or year head of one of the class groups that were being invited to participate, but in some schools it was the Social and Personal Health Education Co-ordinator. In a number of schools, the issues regarding whether or not to participate were discussed at staff meetings or at board of management level, but the procedures within schools were not uniform. Once a school agreed to participate, a date was set for the first research visit.

This main section of the report details the research procedures adopted and the findings. In order to aid clarity, and because the approach adopted was a sequential one with each subsequent phase building on the last, these two sections are integrated. Thus the remainder of the report moves through phases 1, 2 and 3 in that order.

Eighteen schools were invited to participate in this study, 10 in Dublin City and 8 in rural Galway. There were two refusals, both in Dublin. One school was not included because they had too few pupils and no extra workspace *(see Table 2)*. Thus the school level response rate was 83.3%. Two school classes in each school, a total of 16 classrooms, participated in phase 1, 8 groups of children were involved in phase 2, 8 groups in phase 3 and 1 group of young people were involved in the final phase. Thus 33 groups of children and young people aged 8-19 years were included in this study.

TABLE 2: School response rates

LOCATION	SCHOOL TYPE	REFUSAL	NOT APPROPRIATE	ACCEPTANCE
Dublin	Primary	1[1]	-	4
	Post-Primary	1[2]	-	4
Galway	Primary	-	1[3]	4
	Post-Primary	-	-	3[4]

[1] This mixed gender primary school declined to participate on the grounds that they were involved in a myriad of other research activities.

[2] This girls secondary school declined as the principal reported he *"could not see the value of it"* and *"they were already randomly selected for another study"*.

[3] Although the principal and staff of this mixed primary school agreed to participate, there was only one girl in 5th class.

[4] Only 3 schools were required here as the school allocated to take photographs was a co-educational post-primary. In all other groups the photograph phase was undertaken by pupils in single sex schools.

The participating schools reflect the range of public education available in Ireland: small rural primary schools, large urban primary schools, single sex and mixed schools, secondary, vocational and community post-primary schools.

RESEARCH TEAMS

Two research teams were convened for this research. The first comprised of one man and two women, one a qualified and experienced primary school teacher, the others experienced data collectors. They undertook the first phase of this research which involved visiting schools, introducing children to the concept of well-being, distributing cameras and showing children how to use them, collecting used cameras from schools, returning developed photographs to children and facilitating the children in annotating the photographs as to the content and its meaning for them.

The second team comprised one man and one woman, both trained and experienced youth workers with considerable experience of group facilitation and one an experienced researcher. The second team undertook the facilitation of the photograph categorisation, the schema development and the schema integrations. Thus the first team worked on the first phase and the second on the later phases. The process is summarised in Table 3.

TABLE 3: Summary of process

STAGE	SCHOOL VISIT	ACTIVITY
Preparation	Visit	Sample and recruit schools
	Prior to visit	Request and secure parental consent
Phase 1	First set of schools: 1st visit	Request child consent, explain process, distribute cameras
	Between visits	Children take photographs
	First set of schools: 2nd visit	Cameras collected from school
	Between visits	Cameras developed and processed and labels affixed to back of photographs
	First set of schools: 3rd visit: part 1 of session	Developed photographs returned to children, children annotate one set of photographs and return to researchers
	First set of schools: 3rd visit: part 2 of session	Full set of photographs and negatives returned to children
Phase 2	Second set of schools: single visit	Children group pictures together (categorisation) and give the group a title, children give feedback on categories
Phase 3	Third set of schools: single visit part 1 of session	Single sex groups work with examples of the categories to develop patterns (schemata), organise the categories and illustrate schemata with the relationships between categories
	1st visit to new school part 2 of session	Mixed gender group work together to develop a schema representative of the single sex schema
Phase 4	Youth Cafe/Centre: single visit: part 1 of session	Young people work with the developed schemata from phase 3, identifying the similarities and differences between them
	Youth Cafe/Centre: single visit: part 2 of session	Young people work on the development of a schema of well-being to represent all children and young people

Prior to the first school visit (phase 1), schools were sent both letters of information and consent forms for parents. Parents were informed of the study objectives, design and procedures and were requested to complete the consent form, either giving or denying consent for their child to participate. Table 4 *(see page 20)* indicates that of the 332 consent forms distributed, one parental refusal was received (0.3%) and seven children (2.1%) did not return a consent form. As active parental consent was required, these 8 children did not participate in the study. In order to maximise consent for the main study, neither parents nor children were asked to provide consent for the publication of their photographs. Therefore the photographs that illustrate this report were not taken as part of the main study.

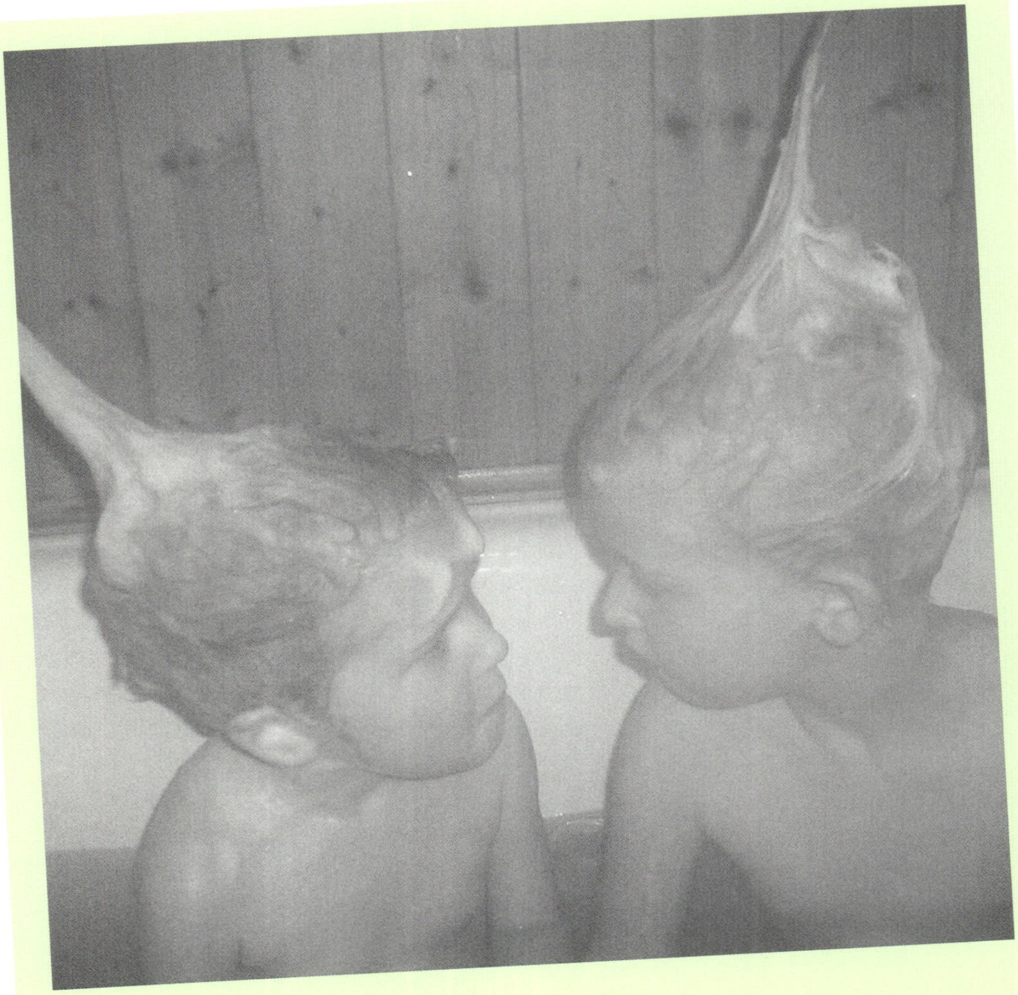

16

17

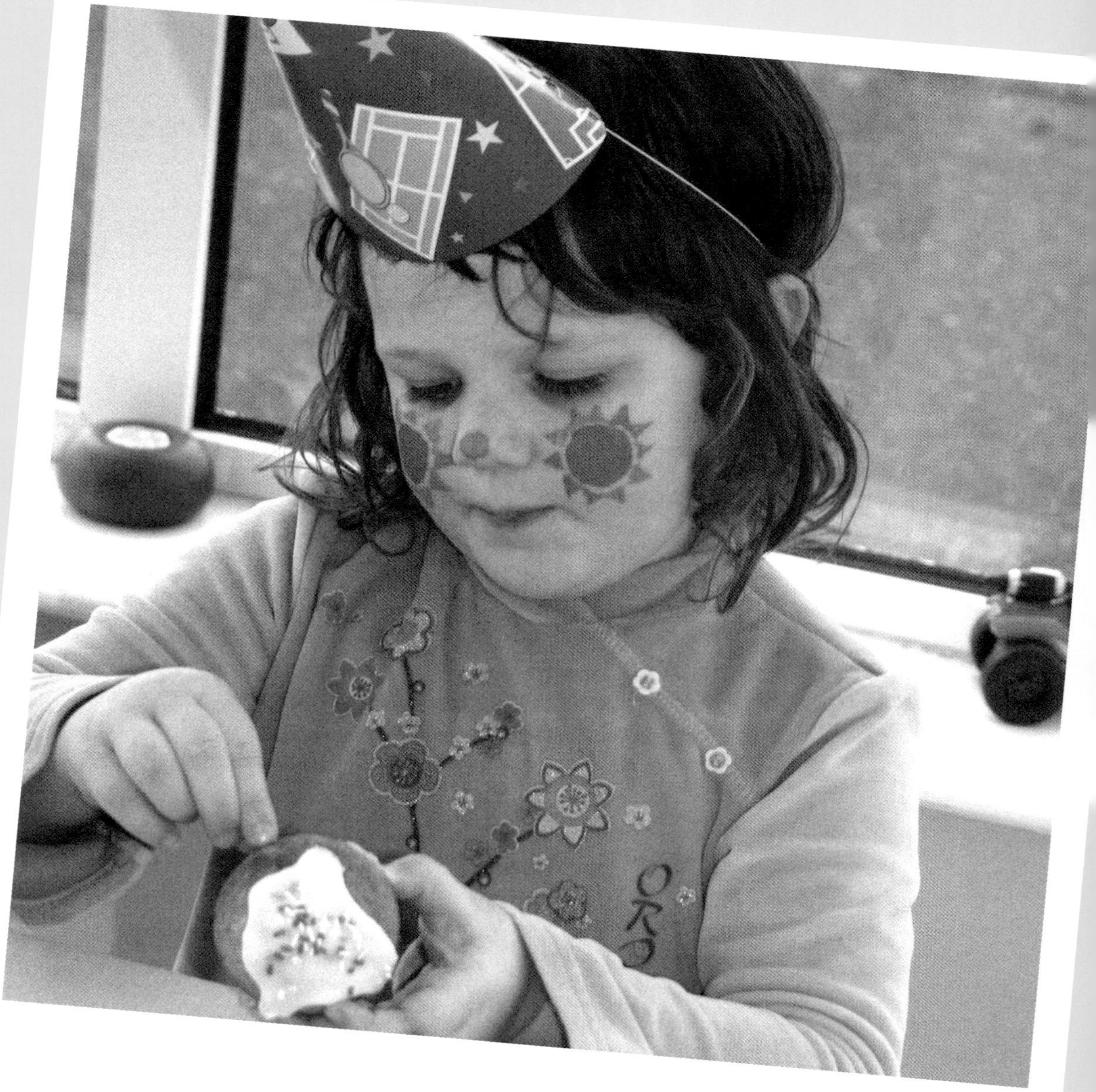

PHASE 1: PHOTOGRAPHING WELL-BEING

This section outlines the procedures involved in the first phase of the research, comprising the visits to the first set of schools to distribute, collect and label the cameras.

INTRODUCING THE CAMERA

The same team of researchers visited every classroom where children were invited to participate in the first phase of this study. The research objectives were to empower children as to their own understanding of well-being, motivate children to participate and to show the children how to use the cameras. First, the researchers collected completed parental consent forms, and in the few cases where a child did not have consent they worked with the teacher to provide an alternative activity. Drawing materials were brought to classrooms and some children drew pictures, but in other cases the teacher organised some reading material for the child.

The purpose of the project was explained to participating children and they were told that their participation was important and could influence what the government does. Children were also told that they did not have to participate and alternative activities were provided, though none took this option. A short introduction to well-being was given in all classrooms. *"Well"* was described as *"feeling good, being happy and able to live your life to the full".* Children were asked to spend some time in quiet reflection on what makes them well and what keeps them well. Subsequently the children were invited to verbalise their suggestions and each suggestion was supported and given positive feedback. If a child was challenged by another because of their suggestion (which happened very rarely), the first child was asked to explain and their answer given support by the research team.

Next, one of the researchers explained how the cameras worked, going through the whole process by taking a photograph. The cameras themselves were distributed to each child and they were asked to write their name, sex and age on the back (e.g. name, boy, 9). With a researcher by their side, children were asked to take a test photograph, with flash, and then shown again how to wind the camera on. At the same time the researchers checked the labeling of the cameras.

Children were reassured that they could take photographs of anything they liked and if they were unable to take a picture of something that they felt should be included (such as a holiday, a grandparent who lives elsewhere or the seaside), then they could take a picture of a photograph or brochure. They were told that they did not have to use all the photographs on the camera, and could take as many pictures as they liked. They were also told that if anyone did not want to take part, that was fine, to just return the camera unused. They were informed as to the date for camera collection and that the researchers would be returning to ask them about the developed photographs. Finally, a letter to parents reinforcing these main procedural points and giving guidelines on how the camera worked was distributed. In many cases the class teacher ensured that the photograph return date was entered into the pupil's homework journal.

RETRIEVING THE CAMERAS FROM CHILDREN

In all cases classroom teachers collected the cameras from the individual children. They were subsequently collected by researchers (Galway) or a courier service (Dublin) and returned to the research centre for processing. In a number of cases cameras were returned late. Where it was possible for these cameras to be processed in time for the third school visit, this was done. Nevertheless all returned cameras were processed. A total of 266 children participated in all stages of this first phase, returning 5,334 photographs.

LABELING PHOTOGRAPHS

Two sets of identical photographs were subsequently developed and processed professionally from each disposable camera. Labels were affixed to the back of one of the sets of pictures. Each label was blank except for a short code to indicate the sex, age, class and school of the child, for example B/9/3/2, indicating a nine-year-old boy in third class of school number 2.

The same group of researchers returned to the classroom to ask the pupils to annotate the pictures. At the beginning of the session, children were given positive feedback regarding the photographs and were told that every child took different photographs and that they were all relevant. One set of photographs was returned to pupils and they were asked to write on labels on the back of each picture what was portrayed and why it made them well. Children were told that if the photograph was a test they could write 'test' or 'T' on the label. It was emphasised that this was a 'quiet activity'. Classroom teachers helped to identify children who needed help in writing and assistance was provided by researchers who moved around the classrooms. Each child was spoken to at least once during this process in order to check that they understood and were not distressed in any way by the activity, and to provide help if required. Once this was complete, pupils were given a full set of their own photographs along with their negatives.

The number of individual steps involved in this first phase of the research increased the potential for attrition. Table 4 illustrates the patterns of attrition experienced.

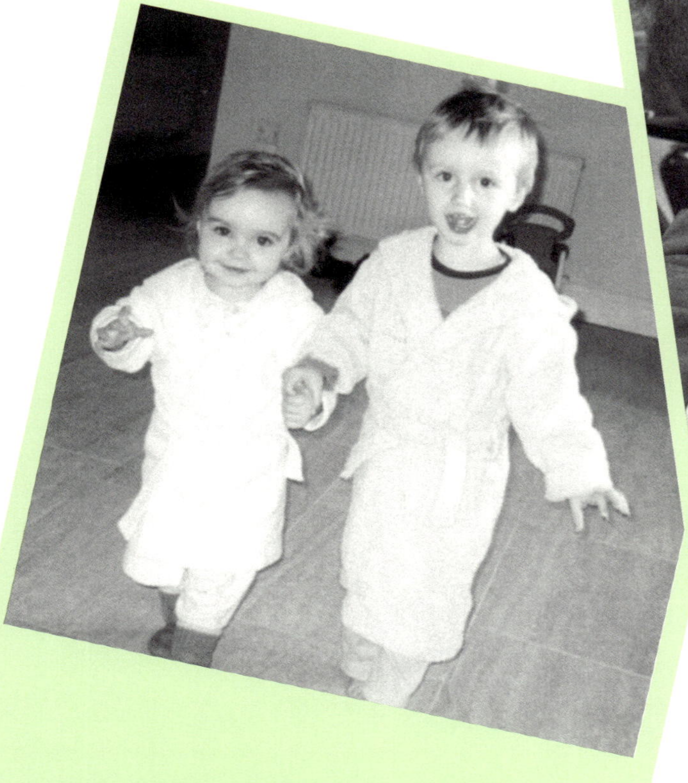

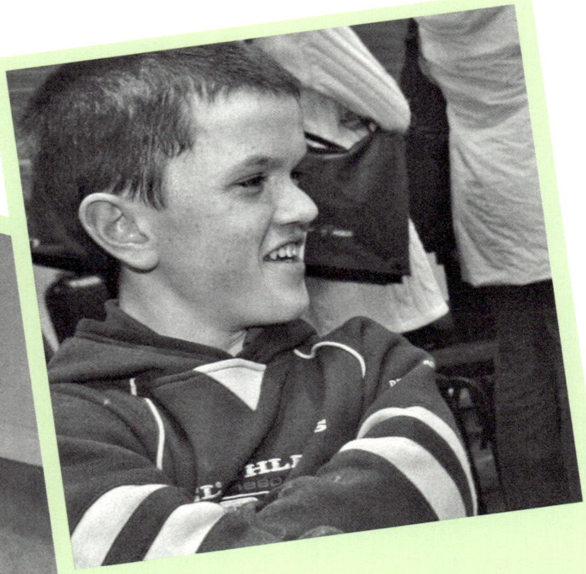

TABLE 4: Sources of attrition

SCHOOL	LEVEL	SCHOOL ROLL	PARENTAL REFUSAL	CONSENT FORMS NOT RETURNED	CHILD REFUSAL	CAMERAS DISTRIBUTED	CAMERAS RETURNED	SETS OF PHOTOS ANNOTATED	ATTRITION	COMMENT
Rural primary girls	Jnr.	14	0	0	0	14	12	12	2	2 cameras returned late
	Snr.	16	0	0	0	16	15	15	1	1 camera returned late
Rural primary boys	Jnr.	17	0	0	0	16	16	16	1	1 absent during camera distribution
	Snr.	11	0	0	0	11	9	9	2	2 cameras returned late
Urban primary girls	Jnr.	18	0	0	0	18	16	16	2	2 cameras returned late
	Snr.	15	0	0	0	15	12	12	3	3 cameras returned late
Urban primary boys	Jnr.	30	0	0	0	27	26	26	4	3 absent during camera distribution 1 camera returned late
	Snr.	27	0	0	0	26	25	20	7	1 absent during camera distribution, 1 camera returned late, 5 absent on day of annotation
Rural post-primary school mixed*	Jnr.	24/30	0/0	2/0	2/7	20/19	15/17	14/6	10/24	2/7 pupil refusals, 2/0 consent forms not returned, 0/4 absent on day of camera distribution, 5/2 cameras returned late, 1/11 absent on day of annotation
	Snr.	17/26	0/0	0/0	0/3	14/21	10/12	10/7	7/19	0/3 pupil refusals, 3/2 absent during camera distribution, 4/9 cameras returned late, 0/5 absent on day of annotation
Urban post-primary school girls	Jnr.	21	0	0	0	20	20	20	1	1 absent when consent forms distributed
	Snr.	16	0	0	0	16	14	14	2	2 cameras not used at all
Urban post-primary school boys	Jnr	27	0	0	0	24	24	24	3	1 pupil refusal, 2 consent forms not returned
	Snr.	24	1	3	0	20	14	13	11	1 parental refusal, 3 consent forms not returned, 6 cameras not returned (including 2 confiscated), 1 absent on day of annotation

* There were clear difficulties with the process in this school. The first time we went through the process the attrition was high, at 10/24 (Jnr.) and 7/17 (Snr.). This meant that the comparability of the data collection was difficult to ascertain. Therefore we returned to the school for another round of the process. However the outcome was worse the second time around, with attrition running at 24/30 (Jnr.) and 19/26 (Snr.). Part of this is due to the heavy involvement in sports in the school, many pupils were absent during visits to the school; either at training or at matches, particularly on the second day of annotation. In the cells for this school the figures are presented x/y, where x is the value for the first round of the process and y for the second. They can be summed to get an overall picture of the school.

REDUCING THE NUMBER OF PHOTOGRAPHS

A member of the research team examined each set of photographs for duplicates (conservatively defined as those with the same picture and the same text). All duplicates were removed from the sets of photographs, as were those labeled 'test' or 'practice', those left blank, those labeled 'nothing', 'mistake', 'error' or 'I didn't mean to take this photograph/picture'. Three photographs were also withdrawn from the process by the research team. Two of the photographs were taken by a single child and the third by a second child. Both of these children were in the same post-primary urban class of boys. All three were withdrawn because of the text on the back of the photographs, which was either homophobic or derogatory regarding another boy in the school. Two of the withdrawn photographs were of the same boy. The research team considered that the risk to the photographed child could be too great if he were to be recognised by other children during the remaining phases of the research. Thus this was considered to be an ethical issue and reinforced the initial decision to involve a separate and unrelated group of children in phases 2 and 3. Table 5 illustrates the numbers and percentages of photographs removed from the initial dataset.

TABLE 5: Photographs removed from the dataset by reason and group (number and % of total photographs taken)

GROUP	BLANK	DUPLICATES	TEST/ PRACTICE	NOTHING	MISTAKE/ ERROR	WITHDRAWN	REMAINING
Rural Primary Girls (n=27)	0 (0.0%)	0 (0.0%)	27 (4.4%)	0 (0.0%)	8 (1.3%)	0 (0.0%)	580 (94.6%)
Rural Primary Boys (n=25)	6 (1.1%)	2 (0.4%)	107 (19.8%)	0 (0.0%)	1 (0.2%)	0 (0.0%)	425 (78.6%)
Urban Primary Girls (n=27)	3 (0.5%)	10 (1.8%)	65 (11.7%)	1 (0.2%)	1 (0.2%)	0 (0.0%)	477 (85.6%)
Urban Primary Boys (n=44)	0 (0.0%)	5 (0.6%)	94 (11.6%)	0 (0.0%)	3 (0.4%)	0 (0.0%)	706 (87.4%)
Rural Post-Primary Girls (n=19)	3 (0.9%)	0 (0.0%)	16 (4.8%)	0 (0.0%)	8 (2.4%)	0 (0.0%)	304 (91.8%)
Rural Post-Primary Boys (n=20)	3 (0.7%)	1 (4.5%)	42 (10.5%)	0 (0.0%)	25 (6.23%)	0 (0.0%)	330 (82.3%)
Urban Post-Primary Girls (n=34)	1 (0.1%)	1 (0.1%)	15 (2.0%)	0 (0.0%)	15 (2.0%)	0 (0.0%)	700 (95.6%)
Urban Post-Primary Boys (n=37)	2 (0.3%)	5 (0.8%)	59 (9.4%)	0 (0.0%)	8 (1.3%)	3 (0.5%)	551 (87.7%)

All remaining photographs were then randomly assigned into groups of 50. This means that each photograph from each child had an equal chance of being employed in later phases of the study.

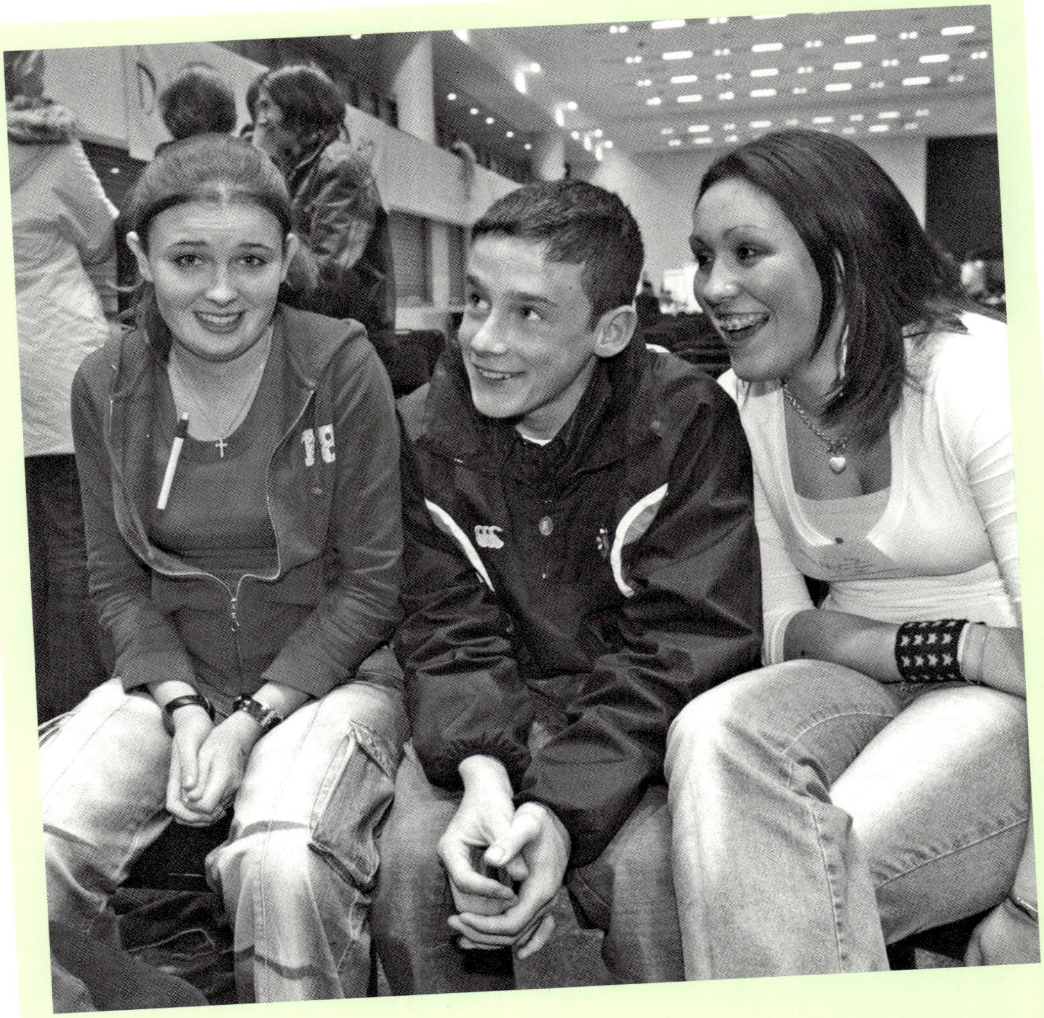

22

23

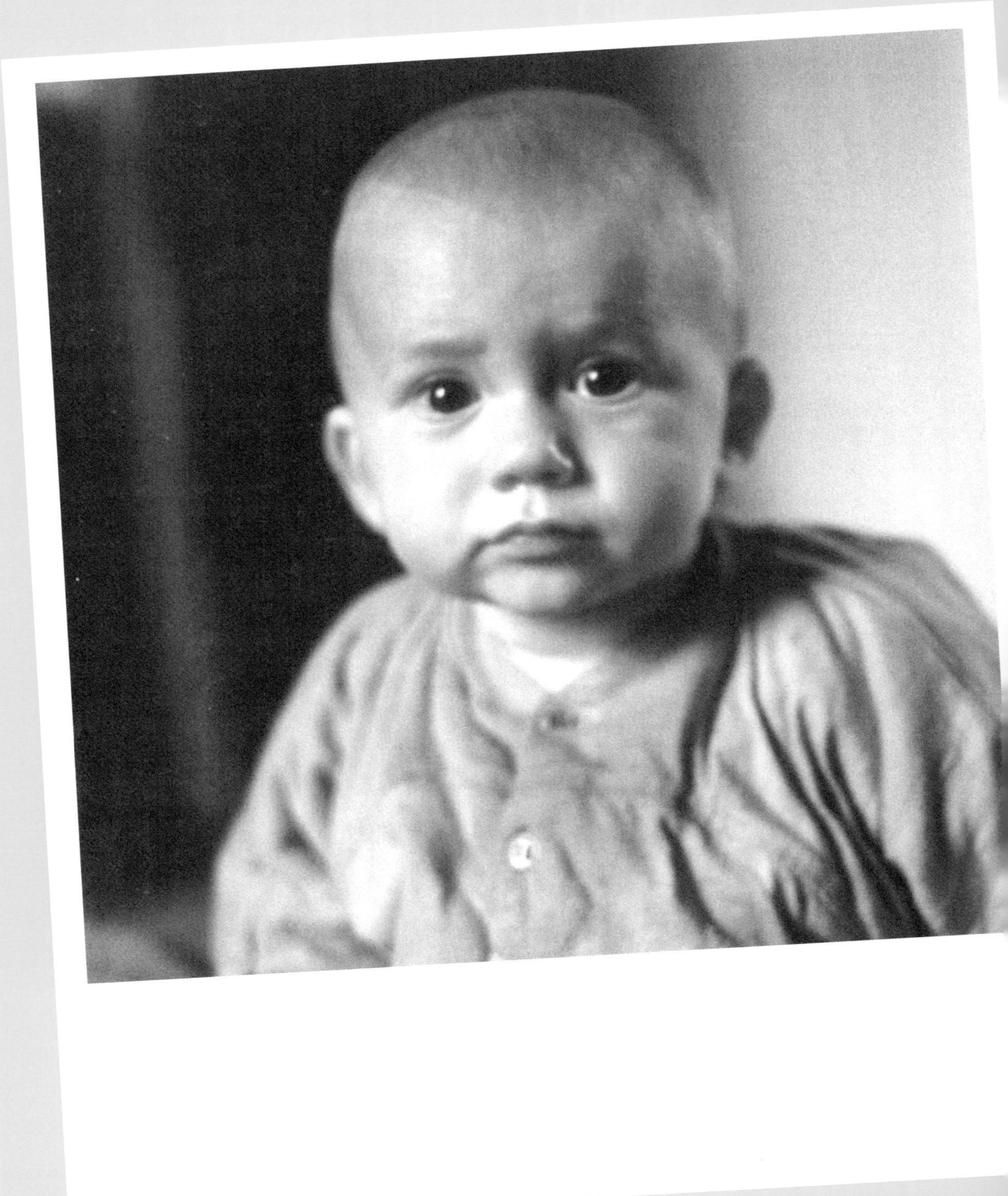

PHASE 2: CATEGORISING THE PHOTOGRAPHS

The second phase involved children who were socio-demographically similar to the photograph-takers, looking at the photographs and dividing them into groups, referred to as categorisation. The task of facilitating this process was undertaken by a second research team who were more experienced in working directly with groups of young people. The objectives for this phase were to have photographs classified into mutually exclusive categories and to agree a title and description for the category.

When researchers visited the schools, they first prepared a group workspace that was outside a formal classroom. When they were joined by each single-sex group of children, each of them, including the researchers, wore a name tag in order to facilitate communication. The group themselves agreed ground rules for the group session, which in all cases included observing confidentiality about the photographs and about the contribution of other group members and showing respect for all group members. By agreement, all sessions were audio-recorded and the researchers took contemporaneous notes. The group was briefly introduced to the concept of well-being, using the same description as was employed in the first phase *(see p. 18)*. They were told that the photographs had been taken by children similar to them and were set the task of devising a categorisation system for the photographs. Sets of 50 photographs were sequentially introduced to the groups. Children decided how many categories there should be, what they should be called and which photographs should be placed in which category. This was an iterative process as children developed categories, divided categories and amalgamated categories throughout. In each case this was achieved by consensus among the children. The researchers continued to introduce sets of 50 photographs until saturation was achieved, that is when no new categories were being created. This took between 200 and 450 photographs, depending on the group. Once the introduction of new sets of photographs ceased, the group concentrated on naming the category and describing it. In most cases the descriptions took the form of listing the content of the photographs. Finally the groups were asked whether there were any relationships between the categories and to discuss whether there were any categories missing. Project managers debriefed researchers after each session.

Tables 6 to 13 demonstrate the numbers and percentages of photographs in each category as determined by the children involved in this phase of the group work process. Under the column 'content/description' the text was provided by the children involved. The final row in each of these tables contains the items or concepts relevant to well-being that the children present said they thought were missing from the photographs.

TABLE 6: The categories of photographs taken and classified by rural primary school girls
(Total number of photographs employed = 250)
(Children's own words are used below)

CATEGORY NAME	CONTENT/DESCRIPTION	NUMBER OF PHOTOS (%)
Friends	All friends together, make me feel happy, play together, make me happy, talks to me, laugh with them, stuff together, when sad they make you happy	73 (29.2%)
Family	Make me feel better when I'm upset, do things for me, look after me, mum buys me clothes, make me feel happy because they are nice, family make me happy, mum makes me feel good because she is funny, family help me learn things, mum and dad take care of me when I'm sick or in bad health	51 (20.4%)
Things to do	Irish dancing shoes, like doing things, swimming fun to do, basketball makes me happy, basketball keeps me healthy, swing makes me happy, running favourite sport, bike - love riding it, exercise, gymnastics makes me happy, wearing/putting on make-up (also added to this category later were: computer - helps me do my homework, music, PS2 fund, instruments make me happy/ fun, computer games, art makes me feel happy because it's pretty	24 (9.6%)
Animals/pets	Horse (friendly), love pets (fish), dogs, cats, playing/cute, horses, sheep, gerbils, make you happy, cuddle them, feeding them, playing with the cats, goldfish (make me happy by swimming), birds	20 (8%)
Houses and rooms	Rooms, bedrooms, bed makes me happy - gives me energy - like sleeping, mum and dad's room, shelters me, fire keeps me warm, very homely, back garden to play in, neighbours house - pretty, new house - exciting	14 (5.6%)
School	Sub-teacher - she is kind, makes (teacher) me feel happy, learning is good, schoolyard - nice to be outside, love seeing my teacher and my friends, class makes me happy, classmates make me happy - love being with them	12 (4.8%)
Researchers	Pictures of researchers, they were nice to me	9 (3.6%)
Toys/teddies	Love them/favourite, fun to play with, make me feel better, hug them, make you happy, had teddy since born - like playing with it	9 (3.6%)
Places	River makes me happy, home (she lives there), beautiful things make her feel well, fish, lake (nice because you can go fishing), USA (likes going there: it's where she's from)	9 (3.6%)
Books	Favourite books, makes me happy, good books - interesting, pass the time, like reading - Harry Potter, when you're bored it's nice to read	7 (2.8%)
Foods	Milk/bread, sweets/coca cola (nice), fruit (like to eat it), mum cooking: makes you feel good because they taste nice, make me really happy	7 (2.8%)
Flowers	Decorated all the room, pretty, make me feel all happy, tell me spring is coming, flowers in my garden	5 (2%)
Churches	Make me feel good, I go there every Sunday, Jesus - he guides me through life, I go to church to speak to God	5 (2%)
Neighbours	Makes me feel happy (nice, friends, comforting), good neighbour, nice	4 (1.6%)
Car	New car (we are getting a new car)	1 (0.4%)
Missing	*Shops - where you buy things that keep you well, Clothes - make you look well, Pony Riding – makes me happy, Hurling/Tennis, Athletics, Pictures of babies, People that help you – doctors/nurses, Electricity (hot shower/bath/ alarms/going to the toilet), Holidays, Getting away, Car - it takes you places*	

TABLE 7: The categories of photographs taken and classified by rural primary school boys
(Total number of photographs employed = 200)
(Children's own words are used below)

CATEGORY NAME	CONTENT/DESCRIPTION	NUMBER OF PHOTOS (%)
Friends	Playing games, make them feel happy, like school because are there, church/ because family there, cool hair/friends, being with them	56 (28%)
Places	Islands/lakes, back gardens/huts, plants/shrubbery, garden, towers, bridges, flowers, trees, makes you feel comfortable, park/water, field, outside	22 (11%)
Pets	Like playing with them, lambs, horses, dogs, cats, cows, ducks, friendly, jump on you	22 (11%)
Soccer and sports	Like football teams, games they play, Gaelic football, makes them happy/play with their friends, things he loves: he plays nearly every day, makes him happy, footballs, fun, soccer goals, stadium/comfortable, Man. Utd. makes him happy, boats make him happy, pitch makes him feel well	18 (9%)
Family	Kind to each other, look out for each other, thinking of each other, love them more than anything in the world, praying for them	18 (9%)
Houses and bedroom	They live there, keep him well, nice place, nice and warm, bring friends/fresh air, kitchen, bedrooms - fun in bedrooms	14 (7%)
TV/Video games	Taken from the fun group	14 (7%)
School/ trophies	Education/friends, my class, classroom makes me happy, the trophy when I scored a goal, school makes me happy	9 (4.5%)
Food	Makes them happy/because you can eat it, favourite food, healthy, sweets/ nice and tasty, fed me, like sweets	5 (2.5%)
Fishing	Fun makes you feel well, fishing rod is very thin	4 (2%)
Fun	Lego, games for fun, bar is fun, bonfire	4 (2%)
Reading	Books and comics I like	3 (1.5%)
Energy/ strength	Bike, allows me to keep going, full of energy	3 (1.5%)
Laughing	Bus driver, funny faces, girls	3 (1.5%)
Trampoline	Is fun	2 (1%)
Clock	-	1 (0.5%)
Cars	-	1 (0.5%)
Arts	-	1 (0.5%)
Missing	*Fruit, Hurling, Rugby, Golf, Running, Exercise, More nature*	

TABLE 8: The categories of photographs taken and classified by urban primary school girls
(Total number of photographs employed = 250)
(Children's own words are used below)

CATEGORY NAME	CONTENT/DESCRIPTION	NUMBER OF PHOTOS (%)
Friends	Happy, best, comfort, loved, amused, play, well	81 (32.4%)
Family	Safe, happy, nice, well, sad, love	47 (18.8%)
Pets/animals	Happy, cuddle, play, love pets	20 (8%)
Environment	Nature, flowers, globe, park	15 (6%)
Playing	Having fun, having a good time	12 (4.8%)
Possessions	Proud, keep amused, poster of favourite pop star, cars	10 (4%)
Art	Happy, proud - best picture, better than someone else, colour	10 (4%)
Teams	Loved playing with others, learn from team	10 (4%)
Teachers	People who teach, like them, teach them, love	8 (3.2%)
Toys	Teddies, dolls, amuse, play love them	7 (2.8%)
Homes	Safe, happy, warm	7 (2.8%)
Places	Life visiting places, cinema, Dublin Castle	6 (2.4%)
Religion	Happy God is there, safe, holy, confirmation	6 (2.4%)
St. Valentine's Day	Happy, show they are loved, show they care	4 (1.6%)
Food	Healthy, delicious	3 (1.2%)
People	Other people	2 (0.8%)
Trophies	Winning, proud	1 (0.4%)
Birthday	Excited, happy	1 (0.4%)
Missing	*School (3 aspects): lively, busy, learning, Clothes: feel happy in the clothes you like, Inside of homes: which room they like the best, People around you: you have to meet people in order to get friends, Sitting in front seat makes you feel older and makes you feel well, Being happy makes you feel well, Could eat good food but be alone and so not be happy and then not be well, Think older kids not into family so much.*	

TABLE 9: The categories of photographs taken and classified by urban primary school boys
(Total number of photographs employed = 200)

CATEGORY NAME	CONTENT/DESCRIPTION	NUMBER OF PHOTOS (%)
People	Friends - being in a team. Family - mothers, fathers, brothers, sisters, grandparents, uncles, aunts	71 (35.5%)
Games	Rugby, Gaelic, soccer, warhammer, computer games, playstations, stickers, skateboarding, gym, trampoline, being in a team, success, swimming, basketball, scoring a goal	68 (34%)
Food and vitamins	Milk, vitamins, vegetables, dinner time, fridge	17 (8.5%)
Animals	Playing with pets, birds, cats, dogs, calf, animal kisses, fish, things you like and things that make you laugh	16 (8%)
Places	People in yard, countryside, globe, home	10 (5%)
Comfort	Relaxing, bed, warmth (sunset and fire)	5 (2.5%)
Plants - oxygen-givers	Flowers, plants, pond, butterflies	5 (2.5%)
Cars	Helps get around to meet friends and other places	3 (1.5%)
Music	*(guitar + CD)*	2 (1%)
Remembering being a baby	*(babies, shoes)*	1 (0.5%)
Books	Reading	1 (0.5%)
Religion	(Child's Bible)	1 (0.5%)
Missing	*Clothes, Trains and Boats – things you love, Things that make you feel good, Medicine, Water, Money, Circuses/Cinema, Christmas, Presents, Scenery, Holidays, Everything relates to life, Plants give you air, Need food to live, Things you like, Learning to expand your vocabulary, Develop minds*	

TABLE 10: The categories of photographs taken and classified by rural post-primary school girls (Total number of photographs employed = 300)
(Children's own words are used below)

CATEGORY NAME	CONTENT/DESCRIPTION	NUMBER OF PHOTOS (%)
Friends	Make you laugh, cheer you up, make you happy	145 (48.3%)
Family	Spending time with them, make you laugh, playing jokes, make you smile	19 (6.3%)
Pets	Keeps me company, playing with them when I'm angry, love animals, sense of independence, give me enjoyment, hobbies/cats/horses	17 (5.7%)
Music	Playing violin, playing piano, fun, choir, things to do, CD player, different music to suit my moods, helps me to forget my problems, keeps me sane, like their music	16 (5.3%)
Sports	Trampoline/hurling/camogie medals, jersey, going to the match, a lot of enjoyment, basketball, football, workouts, exercise	14 (4.7%)
Favourite places	I love playing outside, in the sitting room, friend's house, love the countryside, journey to school, sense of peace and tranquility, quiet	13 (4.3%)
Stuff	Make-up, smelling nice for the lads, confidence, stuff on my bed to sleep in, collecting things, basketball	9 (3%)
TV	Love watching TV, up to date soaps/programmes, makes me happy, watching films/relaxing	8 (2.7%)
Lads you like	Makes me feel very happy, walks me home after school, love him to pieces, like him	8 (2.7%)
Horses	Hobbies/Interests, life, make me happy, get away from things	7 (2.3%)
Beds and Bedrooms		6 (2%)
Food	Cheers me up, keeps me well, hate the feel of hunger	3 (1%)
Houses	Shelter/sense of security, love my house, I like spending time there	3 (1%)
Phones	Contact with friends, like my best friend	3 (1%)
Clothes	Love shopping/gives me confidence/feel better about myself	3 (1%)
Cars	My love of cars/travelling	3 (1%)
Computers & Playstation	-	3 (1%)
Art	Art – favourite subject, teacher is an inspiration to me	3 (1%)
Teddies	I have had them since I was a baby, cheer me up when I'm feeling down	2 (0.7%)
Fags	Smoking: Keeps me happy when I'm in a bad mood, bad side to health	2 (0.7%)
Bus/bus driver	-	2 (0.7%)
Trophies/ medals	-	2 (0.7%)
Bad days	Need bad days to appreciate the good ones, tests	2 (0.7%)
Money	Need money for clothes and to go to discos	2 (0.7%)
Foróige club	-	1 (0.3%)
Teachers	-	1 (0.3%)
Children/ babysit	-	1 (0.3%)
Photographs/ happy memories	-	1 (0.3%)
Magazines	-	1 (0.3%)
Missing	*Beach, Sunny weather, Discos – enjoying self, keep you happy, getting excited, fun with friends, Pool, Cinema, Shopping – music, clothes, make-up*	

TABLE 11: The categories of photographs taken and classified by rural post-primary school boys (Total number of photographs employed = 300)
(Children's own words are used below)

CATEGORY NAME	CONTENT/DESCRIPTION	NUMBER OF PHOTOS (%)
Friends	Funny, make me feel good	110 (36.7%)
Sports	Soccer/pool/hurling, snooker, GAA, rugby, pitches, swingball, hurly	21 (7.1%)
Music & moshers	Guitars, amps, music posters, music sheets	19 (6.3%)
Family	Grandads/Grandmas	17 (5.7%)
TV	Ireland beating England, watching TV, entertained, interesting	14 (4.7%)
Dogs	Pets/dogs	11 (3.7%)
Cars	They like their cars fast, I like reading about cars, their cars, car magazines	10 (3.3%)
Computers	Pictures of computers	9 (3.0%)
Food & drinks	Can't smile without food, food's good for you, can't live without food	9 (3.0%)
Music systems	Amps, stereo systems	8 (2.7%)
Houses	Sitting rooms, where I live	8 (2.7%)
Sheep	Give me money when sold, pets	8 (2.7%)
Hobbies	-	7 (2.3%)
Phones	Mobile phones, texting, contacting	6 (2.0%)
Playstations	Occupied, fun	6 (2.0%)
*School	-	5 (1.7%)
Football teams	-	4 (1.3%)
Countryside	Scenery	3 (1.0%)
Community centres	-	2 (0.7%)
Money	Buy sweets/food, money from working with people	2 (0.7%)
Clothes	-	2 (0.7%)
Bedrooms	-	2 (0.7%)
Fire and water	-	2 (0.7%)
Sheds	Farming and helping father	2 (0.7%)
Traveling	-	2 (0.7%)
*Trophies	-	2 (0.7%)
Pubs	-	2 (0.7%)
Looks	Tattoo	1 (0.3%)
Aftershave	-	1 (0.3%)
Sky	-	1 (0.3%)
Bikes	-	1 (0.3%)
Boiling water	-	1 (0.3%)
*Reading	-	1 (0.3%)
Medicine	-	1 (0.3%)
Missing	*Simpsons, Entertainment (cinema, theatre, discos, concerts)*	

TABLE 12: The categories of photographs taken and classified by urban post-primary school girls (Total number of photographs employed = 450)
(Children's own words are used below)

CATEGORY NAME	CONTENT/DESCRIPTION	NUMBER OF PHOTOS (%)
Best friends	Always there for me, good mates, make me feel good, make me laugh, cheer me up, make me feel good, make me happy, spend time with them	144 (32.0%)
Family	My fav sisters, dad/mam love them, loving sister/auntie, make me laugh, make me happy, brother make me smile, love them	86 (19.1%)
School friends	The gang, laughing/new friends, kind/sound, nice/sense of humour, fun, makes me happy to be with my friends, great friend, enjoy myself	85 (18.9%)
Music	Makes me feel good (concert ticket), love music, helps me to study, fav groups, Busted concert	16 (3.6%)
Sport	Camogie, basketball, enjoy playing, keeps me sane, love football, watching teams play, hockey (like playing), skateboarding (on-line skating), managers guide me, baseball, Tae Kwando, Dublin Jersey	15 (3.3%)
Pets	Cats/dogs, my dog is good for a hug, pets do funny things, fun to play with, very cute, crazy cats, being with them	14 (3.1%)
Junk/nice food	MacDonalds, junk food, wheetos make me happy, love chocolates, fruit, eating makes me happy, addicted to coke, love food, take-aways are great	14 (3.1%)
Stuff; make-up, phones, magazines, etc.	Money, spending money on phone, make-up, communication with phone, hair straighteners, hair products, smelling nice, chain belonging to granny	9 (2.0%)
Guys	He is gorgeous, makes me feel good, love him, makes me happy/can trust him, cheers me up	8 (1.8%)
Memories	Den TV, T-shirts, I'm important, candles make me calm when I'm stressed	6 (1.3%)
Computers/ TV, etc.	Love watching TV when I'm stressed, computers (I use for school), I keep in touch by e-mail, x-box, I enjoy playing internet chatting to friend	6 (1.3%)
Phones	Communication with friends – the best	5 (1.1%)
Outside	Flowers, love being outside, the sun, airplane reminds me about holidays	5 (1.1%)
PJs and beds	Love sleep, relaxed, beds, need to sleep, warm	4 (0.9%)
Hobbies	Music instrument, Irish dancing, shopping	4 (0.9%)
Entertainment	Break from reality, comedy, Grease film, love comedy	4 (0.9%)
Shoes/clothes	Everybody needs clothes	3 0.7%)
Religion	Keep hold of religion/pastor teaches the bible	3 (0.7%)
Me	Picture of themselves being themselves, love being themselves	3 (0.7%)
Houses and streets	I love my house, I love living there	3 (0.7%)
Special occasions	Christmas, birthday, to be with family	2 (0.4%)
Light & water	Keeps my thirst quenched	2 (0.4%)
Children	Cute – love them	2 (0.4%)
Books	Love reading/politics	2 (0.4%)
Culture		1 (0.2%)
Cranky	Someone in a bad mood	1 (0.2%)
Charity	Giving money to the poor	1 (0.2%)
Cars		1 (0.2%)
Art	Appreciate the area around me	1 (0.2%)
Missing	*Ross O'Carroll Kelly books, Magazines, More comical/funny things, More taking it easy, Karaoke machine, Sleep-overs, Shops, Places you like e.g. Stephen's Green, Spire, More beds and snuggling up in big chairs and cushions, More memories – of good times, Doing stupid stuff and laughing, Pictures of school – canteen, grounds, boys playing football, More music – bands, Pool/snooker, More MacDonalds*	

TABLE 13: The categories of photographs taken and classified by urban post-primary school boys (Total number of photographs employed = 350)
(Children's own words are used below)

CATEGORY NAME	CONTENT/DESCRIPTION	NUMBER OF PHOTOS (%)
Friends	Make them feel happy, good, sit beside them	88 (25.1%)
Technology	Computers, TV makes me happy, playstation, Simpsons	45 (12.9%)
School	Like school, classmates, teachers	23 (6.6%)
Playing sports	Sports gear, playing sports	23 (6.6%)
Music	Listening to music, stereos, album, collection of CDs, bringing music wherever they go, walkmans, guitar, keeps me occupied, concerts, drums/keyboard	21 (6.0%)
Pets	Cats/dogs, to play with, companionship, fun, stops you getting bored, cheering up	18 (5.1%)
Places	Surroundings, makes me happy, skating, fresh air, do things that they like	17 (4.9%)
Hostages (family)	Cousins, babies/mothers, fathers/brothers and sisters	17 (4.9%)
Food	Kitchen, I love to cook, coke/pizza, fries, bread, no pictures of good food	14 (4.0%)
Cars & crap	They like, they give pleasure	12 (3.4%)
Mobile phones	Make me happy, talk to their friends	11 (3.1%)
Watching/ following sports	Man United	11 (3.1%)
Gardens	Do gardening work, back garden flowers, makes me happy	9 (2.6%)
People's houses	Warm, safe	7 (2.0%)
Bikes	Transport, love to cycle, go places to cheer me up	6 (1.7%)
Rooms	Comfortable beside fire, bedroom, sleep makes me feel great	5 (1.4%)
Travel	Fun to go somewhere, holidays/skiing	5 (1.4%)
Achievements	Things that make me feel proud	4 (1.1%)
Books	Reading, feeling good	4 (1.1%)
Self-consciously ironic abstract photography*	-	3 (0.9%)
Sexy photos	-	2 (0.6%)
Money*	Poor little rich boys	2 (0.6%)
Models*	-	2 (0.6%)
Trees*	-	1 (0.3%)
Miscellaneous	Don't know why	
Missing	*Drink and drugs, More outside school, I love stairs, Stuff made selves, Bands they like, Doing stuff they like, Pictures of girls, Fruit tarts makes you happy, Eating apples makes me happy*	

* combined by the group of children to make the category 'miscellaneous'

Table 14 provides a summary of the categorisation process. For each group of children all categories with more than 5% of the photographs are included among the categories listed in the first column. In some groups the category names employed by the children were not exactly the same and thus this table must be interpreted with due care. For example, for the rural primary school girls, the percentage given for 'environment/places' includes 2% for 'flowers' as these are mentioned by other groups as being part of the 'environment' category. Even with this proviso in mind, the percentages of the photographs from each group that these ten categories account for is substantial, ranging from 89.0% to 76.4%.

TABLE 14: Summary of categorisation phase: percentages of photographs by group and category

CATEGORY	PRIMARY				POST-PRIMARY				MEAN
LOCATION	RURAL		URBAN		RURAL		URBAN		ALL
GENDER	GIRLS	BOYS	GIRLS	BOYS	GIRLS	BOYS	GIRLS	BOYS	ALL
Friends	29.2	28.0	32.4	17.8	48.3	36.7	50.9	25.1	33.55
Family	20.4	9.0	18.8	17.8	6.3	5.7	19.1	4.9	12.75
Sport/teams	3.2	9.0	4.0	17.0	4.7	7.1	3.3	9.7	7.25
Pets/animals	8.0	11.0	8.0	8.0	5.7	6.4	3.1	5.1	6.91
Environment/ places	5.6	11.0	6.0	7.5	4.3	1.0	1.1	7.5	5.50
TV/Video games	3.2	7.0	-	-	3.7	7.7	1.3	12.9	4.48
Homes/houses	5.6	7.0	2.8	2.5	3.0	3.4	0.7	2.0	3.38
Food	2.8	2.5	1.2	8.5	1.0	3.0	3.1	4.0	3.26
Music	3.2	-	-	1.0	5.3	6.3	3.6	6.0	3.17
School/teachers	4.8	4.5	3.2	-	0.3	1.7	-	6.6	2.64
TOTALS	86.0	89.0	76.4	80.1	82.6	79.0	86.2	83.8	82.89

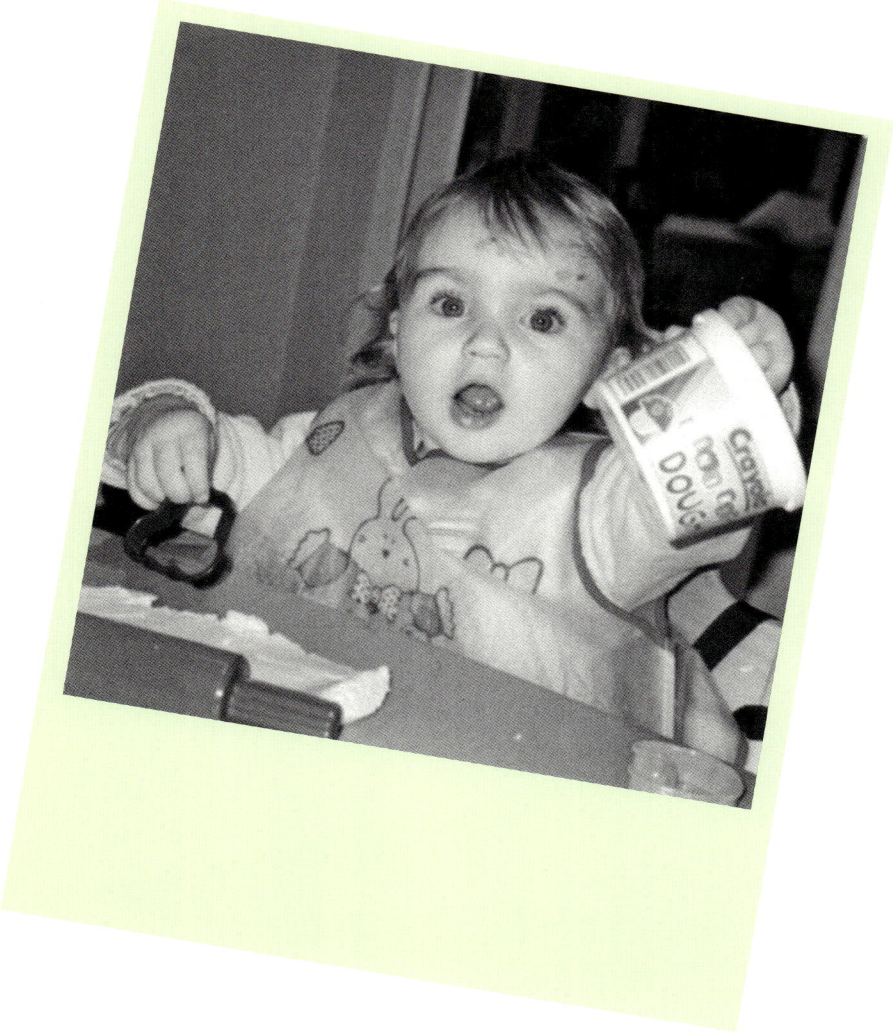

33

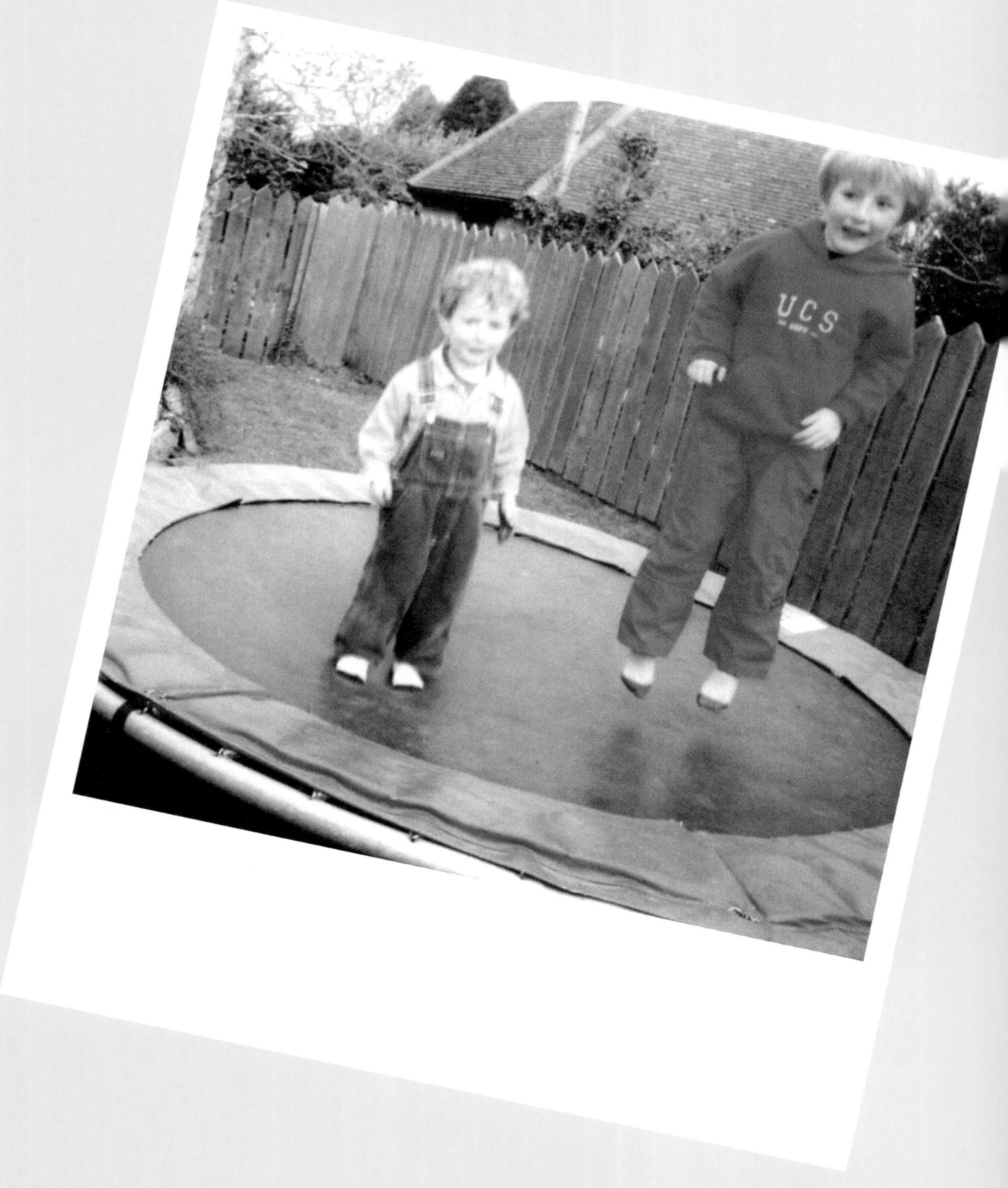

PHASE 3: DEVELOPING SCHEMATA OF WELL-BEING

Following the photograph categorisation, a label with the derived category name was attached to a sample photograph from each category. Care was taken to choose photographs that were most similar to the remainder of the category and which were unambiguous. In each case this was conducted by a single senior researcher. A second set of category names was also prepared on flashcards. Finally a number of blank flashcards were prepared. The labeled photographs, labeled and blank flashcards were brought to the schema development group sessions, along with coloured A1 paper, markers, blu-tak, sellotape and stickies.

The set-up stages of the schema development mirrored those for the photograph categorisation phase. The same pair of researchers visited schools, prepared the workspace, distributed name tags, agreed ground rules with the children and introduced the concept of well-being. Then the children were divided by sex: the female researcher worked with the girls and the male researcher with the boys. In both groups the photography and photograph categorisation phases were explained. In each group the children were shown the sets of labeled photographs that had been taken and categorised by children who were socio-demographically similar to them. Thus the post-primary urban boys were shown the labeled photographs based on the categories developed by post-primary urban boys from photographs taken by post-primary urban boys, and so on. The children were invited to look at the labeled photographs and to think about how they could be arranged or organised into a pattern onto the A1 sheets of card. They were not asked to order them in any way or to place them in a hierarchy. In all groups two sheets of A1 card were required to adequately represent the categories and these were sellotaped together. The placement of the photographs engendered considerable discussion about the categories and their relationships with each other. The groups were told that they did not have to use all the categories/photographs and could merge or amalgamate categories if they felt that was appropriate. They were also given the opportunity to add new categories and place them on the schema. The blank flashcards were used for this purpose. Finally the groups were asked to indicate on their schema which of the categories were related to each other and this was achieved by using markers to draw arrows on the schema itself.

Next, the groups of boys and girls were brought together and this part of the group session was co-facilitated by both researchers. They were shown both gender-specific schemata and asked to develop a third schema that would represent both boys and girls. For this exercise they were asked to use the flashcards with the category names. In most cases the mixed group took the same approach to this as they had done in their gender-specific groups. They decided which categories should be placed together or merged while at the same time deciding on a pattern, placed and secured the labeled flashcards onto the coloured A1 sheets of card, and if relevant to their schema, drew arrows linking the categories.

All sessions were audio-recorded and the researchers took contemporaneous notes. Project managers debriefed researchers after each session. These data are employed in the interpretation of the schema and to highlight issues that arose during the course of schema development.

This next section presents the schemata developed by the groups of children. In the figures below an attempt has been made to be as faithful as possible to the schemata developed. The categories are named as they were by the children and placed relative to other categories as they appeared on the sheets of A1 card. Some schemata need to be viewed from a landscape position and this reflects the way that the children taped together the sheets of A1. Two sorts of arrow are employed in these schemata: the first open type arrow (⟶) indicates relationships between categories which are either unidirectional (⟶) or bidirectional (⟷). The second type of arrow, found on fewer schemata are closed arrows (⟶) and are used to indicate the direction of flow (usually from most important to less important). In some schemata the children have numbered the categories and the meaning of this for a given schema is given in the accompanying text. Finally within the schemata, the font size used for the category name is designed to reflect the original size of that category from phase 2, the photograph categorisation stage. Thus categories that originally comprised 10% of the original set of pictures are represented here in font size 12. The legend used to apply this is given in Table 15.

TABLE 15: Percentage photographs in original category and corresponding font size in schemata

%	FONT SIZE
Less than 2%	8
2-6%	10
7-14%	12
15-24%	14
25-35%	16

Given the degree of removal of the joint schema construction from the original photographs, all the category names in the joint schemata are in 12 point.

In some cases, children merged or amalgamated categories, and where this happened it is detailed in the text and the new category name has been entered into the schema in **bold** font. Where children have added completely new categories, this is also written in the text and is represented on the schema by having the category name *italicised*. In the body of the text, italics indicate direct quotes from the children.

RURAL PRIMARY SCHOOL GIRLS

This first schema (Figure 1), illustrates the complexity with which children view the connections between aspects of their well-being. It can be read from top to bottom in terms of importance, so that 'family' (closely followed by 'animals and pets') was considered the most important and 'school' least important for well-being. Only one category from the original categorisation phase, that of 'researcher', was not employed by this group in the construction of their schema. The category 'friends' emerges as the most connected aspect. Also of note is the category 'old car' that was perceived as enabling or facilitating many of the other aspects of well-being. Two categories stand alone, 'books' and 'flowers', although they were not considered least important. 'Toys and teddies' were placed relatively low within the hierarchy, and were considered as childish by these 5th and 6th class pupils. Only one relationship was seen as bidirectional, that between 'family' and 'houses and rooms'.

FIGURE 1: Rural Primary School Girls

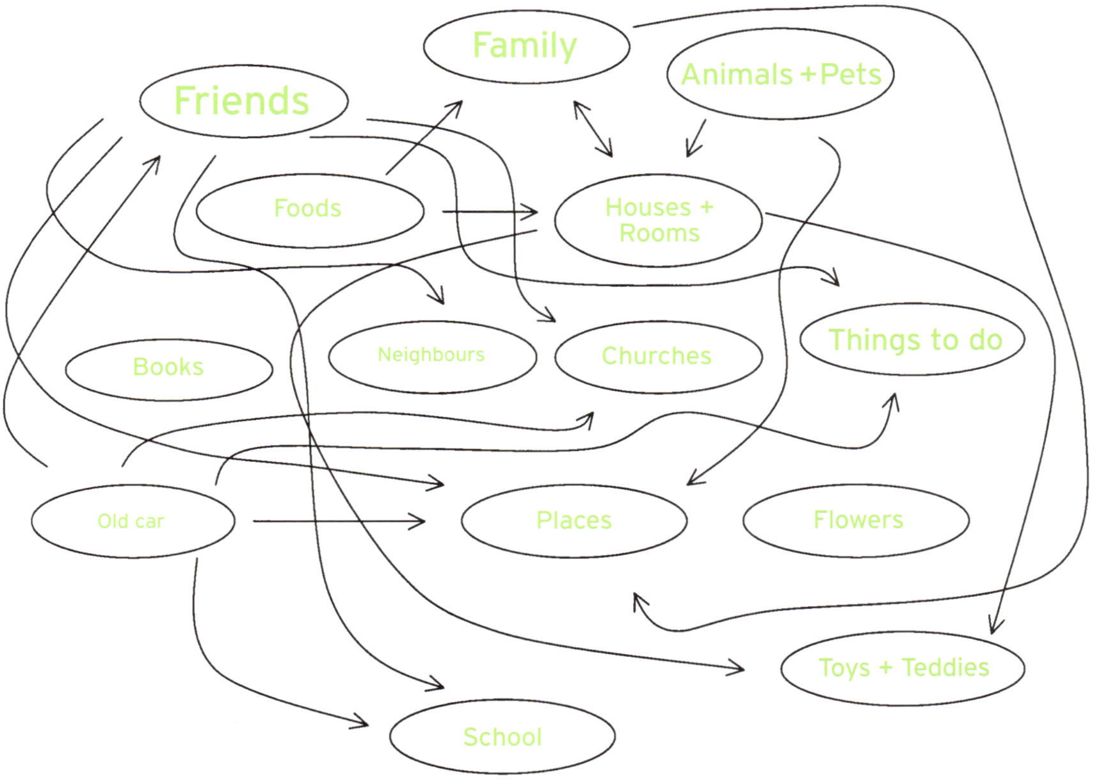

RURAL PRIMARY SCHOOL BOYS

The categories in this schema (Figure 2) are numbered by importance and characterised by a spiral, where the category 1 ('family') was judged most important and the category 18 ('art') was judged least important. The solid arrows around the outside of the schema represent the spiral. The open arrows between categories represent relationships between categories. Each of these relationships is bidirectional, with only one exception, that from 'soccer and sport' to 'friends', suggesting that these boys make or meet friends through sporting activities. The most connected category is 'friends' linking with 5 categories ('food', 'fun', 'art', 'soccer and sport', and 'video games and TV'), followed by 'house and bedrooms' linking with 5 categories ('family', 'reading', 'clock', 'video games and TV' and 'food'). Three categories were considered to be unconnected ('trampoline', 'fishing', and 'laughing').

FIGURE 2: Rural Primary School Boys

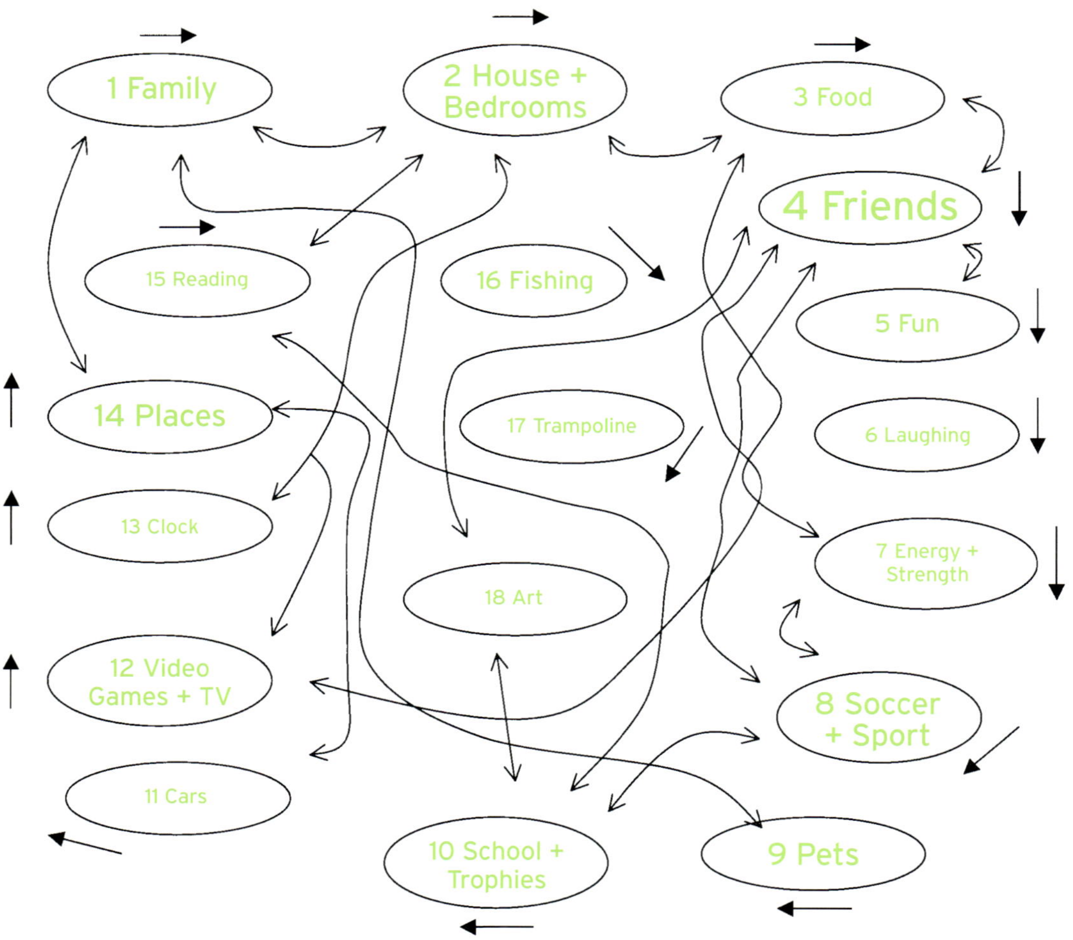

JOINT RURAL PRIMARY SCHOOL

From the original boys 'schema' the only category missing is 'reading', but this is represented in the category 'books'. From the original girls 'schema' the category 'music' is not included here. Two new categories are added to the joint schema (Figure 3); 'holidays' and 'farming'. Although 'holidays' is only connected to the category 'family', 'farming' is connected to 'fun', 'food' and 'things to do'. This reflects the predominantly farming community that the children come from.

This joint schema is constructed in a similar hierarchical fashion to that of the rural primary school girls, running from the top (indicating 'family' as most important) to the bottom ('flowers' and 'clock' are joint least important). The most connected category is 'fun' with 9 connections ('farming', 'family', 'things to do', 'toys and teddies', 'trampoline', 'friends', 'soccer and sports', 'energy and strength', and 'art'), followed closely by 'things to do' with 8 connections ('farming', 'fun', 'cars', 'video games and TV', 'books', 'fishing', 'toys and teddies', and 'art'). This indicates the focus on activity rather than the people present during the activity.

Nevertheless, these children place their families first, as most important. Both 'family' and 'friends' are well connected (4 each). This joint schema confirms the importance of cars as a source of transport, which facilitates other activities.

During the construction of this schema, although the boys and girls agreed on the placement of 'family', the girls argued that 'pets/animals' were only marginally less important. In response the boys insisted that 'soccer and sports' be placed equivalently within the hierarchy, at the same level as 'pets/animals'. This is particularly noteworthy because when the boys had been working on their own schema, they had placed 'soccer and sports' eighth out of eighteen, immediately before 'pets', but below almost all the categories on the next two levels.

FIGURE 3: Joint Rural Primary School

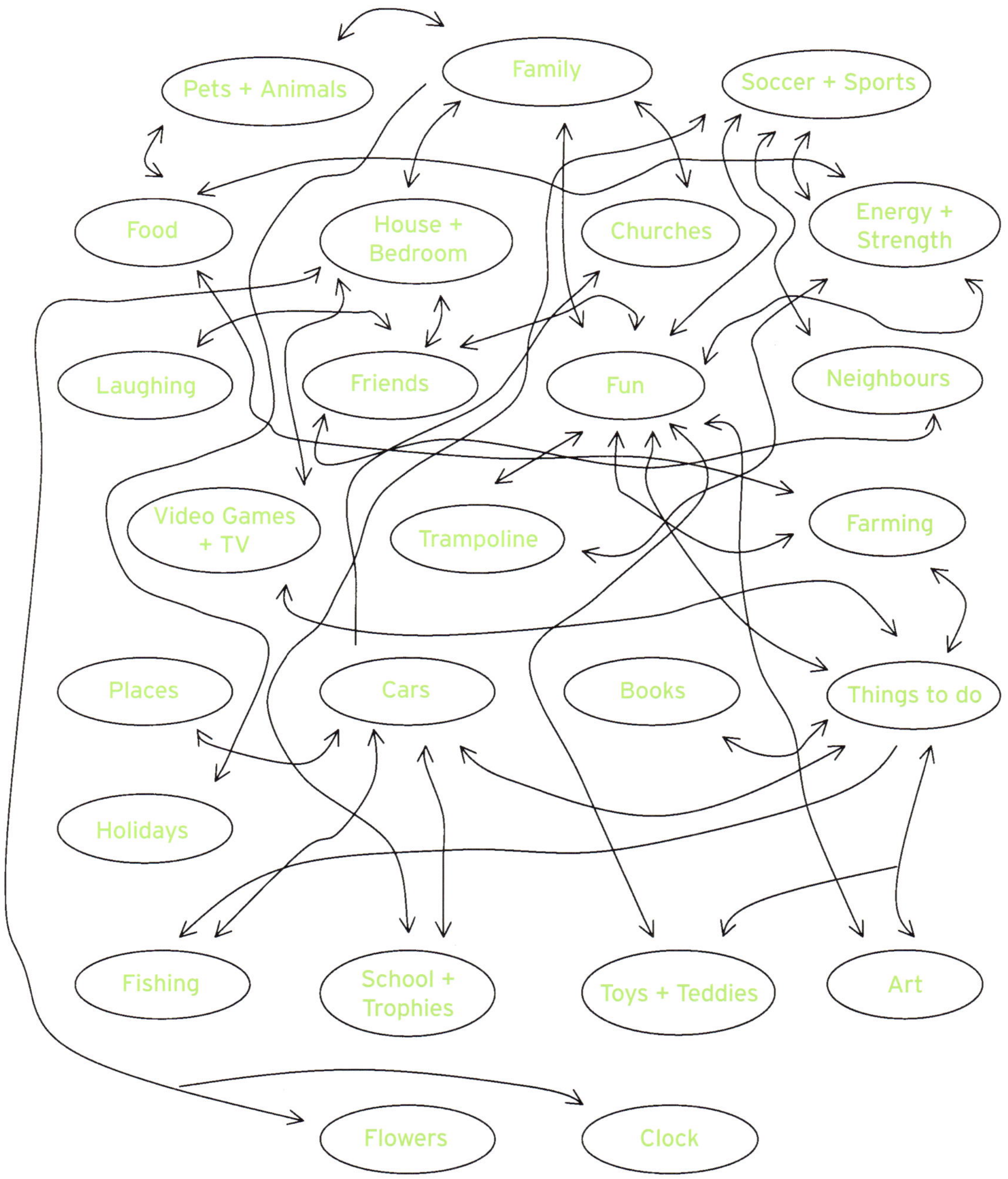

URBAN PRIMARY SCHOOL GIRLS

These girls initially merged 'toys' and 'playing' to make a joint category. In addition, three sets of pairs are placed together: 'possessions' with 'homes', 'places' with 'environment', 'family' with 'pets/animals'. The girls added the categories 'Christmas or other religious celebrations' and 'medicine'. 'Medicine' was described as helping you to get better if you are sick. 'Friends' is the most connected category (connected to 'people', 'teams', 'toys and playing', 'birthday' and 'family') and 'medicine' is the least connected (to 'environment' only). However, the girls reported that all the categories were related to one another.

There was considerable discussion regarding the category 'possessions', 'music' and 'books', which were considered to be part of 'possessions' as were 'pets'. The category itself was placed with 'home', since that is where your 'possessions' are located. Two other issues arose: 'possessions' were characterised as being part of you, *"things you own and control"* and *"things you own and love"*. Secondly, the girls discussed the importance of 'possessions' as indicative of identity, *"you know who you are by what kind of music/toys you have"*.

The girls initially set out to design this schema (Figure 4) as a web. At the centre of the web is the 'family' and the remaining categories were to be placed on the spindles of the web. The web was to be underlaid following the placement of the categories. However, they were placed in no particular order. After the girls started to draw the connections between categories, they realised that their web concept would not be clear or as attractive as they had initially intended, at which point they abandoned the idea of the web. Instead, they decided to number the categories in order of importance for well-being. Numbers 5a and 6a were skipped during the initial stages of the numbering, so rather than re-number every category, they decided that 5a ('toys') should be placed between 'possessions' and 'birthday' and that 6a ('playing') between 'birthday' and 'people'.

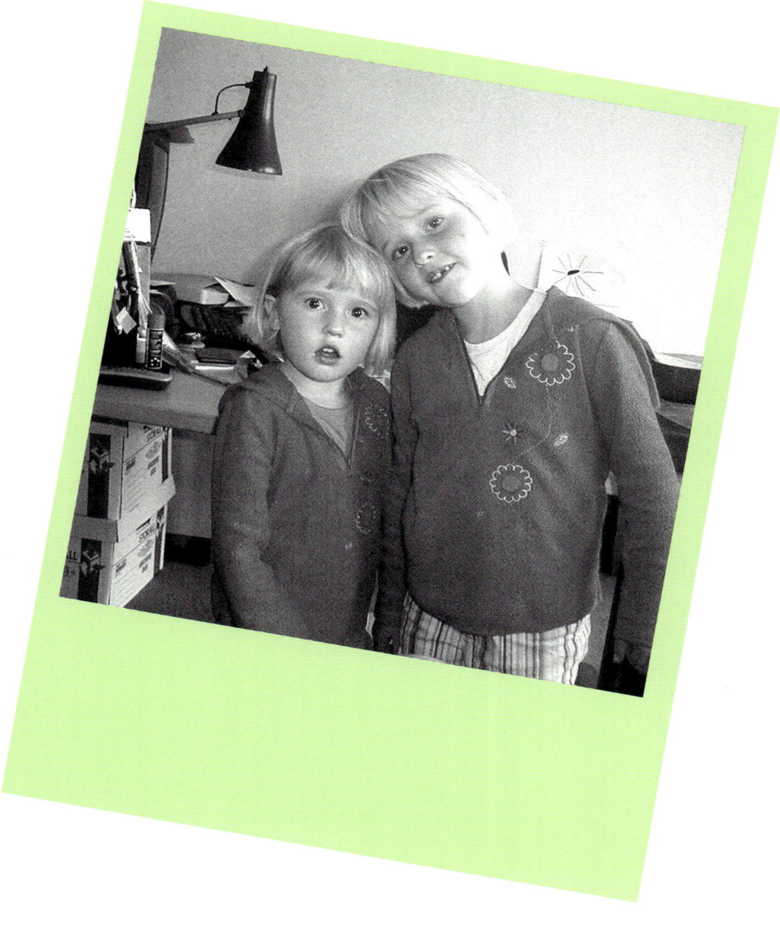

FIGURE 4: Urban Primary School Girls

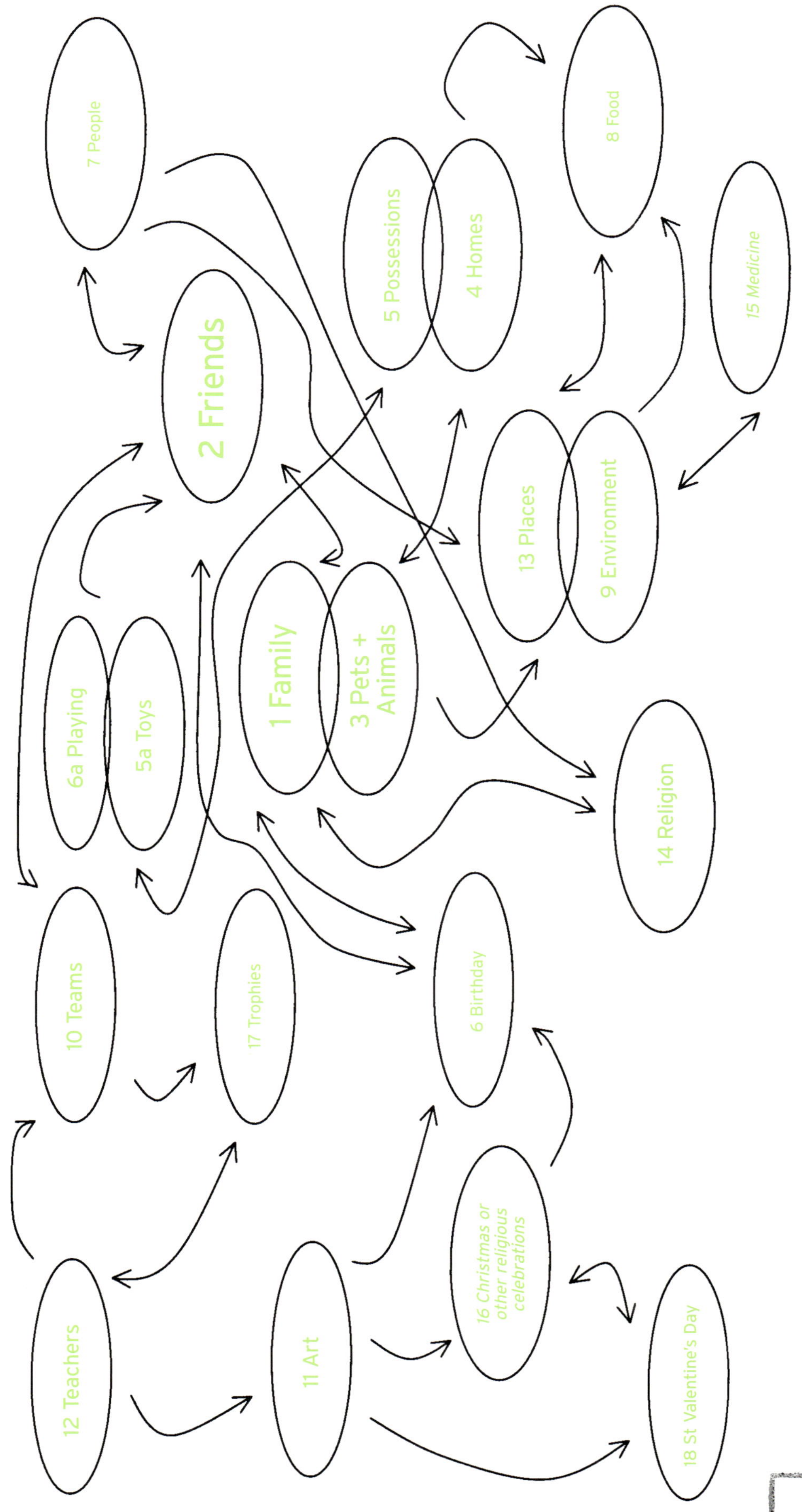

URBAN PRIMARY SCHOOL BOYS

The boys added two new categories: 'TV' and 'holidays'. They placed 'TV' with 'books' (as activities) and 'holidays' with 'places' (as locations), and replaced the category 'remembering being a baby' with the more generic category 'memories'. They also added 'family' and 'friends' to the bottom of the schema (Figure 5), although they were also included in the 'people' category. It should be remembered here that the category 'games' is primarily comprised of sport and also includes some other activities (e.g. collecting stickers, computer games).

The boys organised the categories to appear like a face, with 'games' and 'people' as the eyes, 'religion' and 'cars' as the ears, and so on. They arrived at and agreed this idea very quickly during their schema development session. The categories are also numbered in order of importance, where the category 'people' is labeled 1 as the most important to well-being and 'religion' is labeled 11 as least important. The two sections of the nose, 'food' and 'animals', are jointly labeled as 3, while the categories added by the boys, 'TV', 'holidays', 'family' and 'friends', are not labeled as to their relative importance, indicating that they are perceived as extensions of existing categories rather than being completely original. The boys recognised that both 'family' and 'friends' were included in the original category 'people', but they deliberately placed them on the schema to represent a small beard or *"smig"*.

The most connected category here is 'people': it is connected to 8 other categories ('games', 'cars', 'food', 'memories', 'books', 'plants and oxygen-givers', 'places', and 'music'). In addition, 'family' is connected to 'TV' and 'friends' to 'music'. No category is unconnected, but 'religion', 'comfort' and 'memories' have a single connection each.

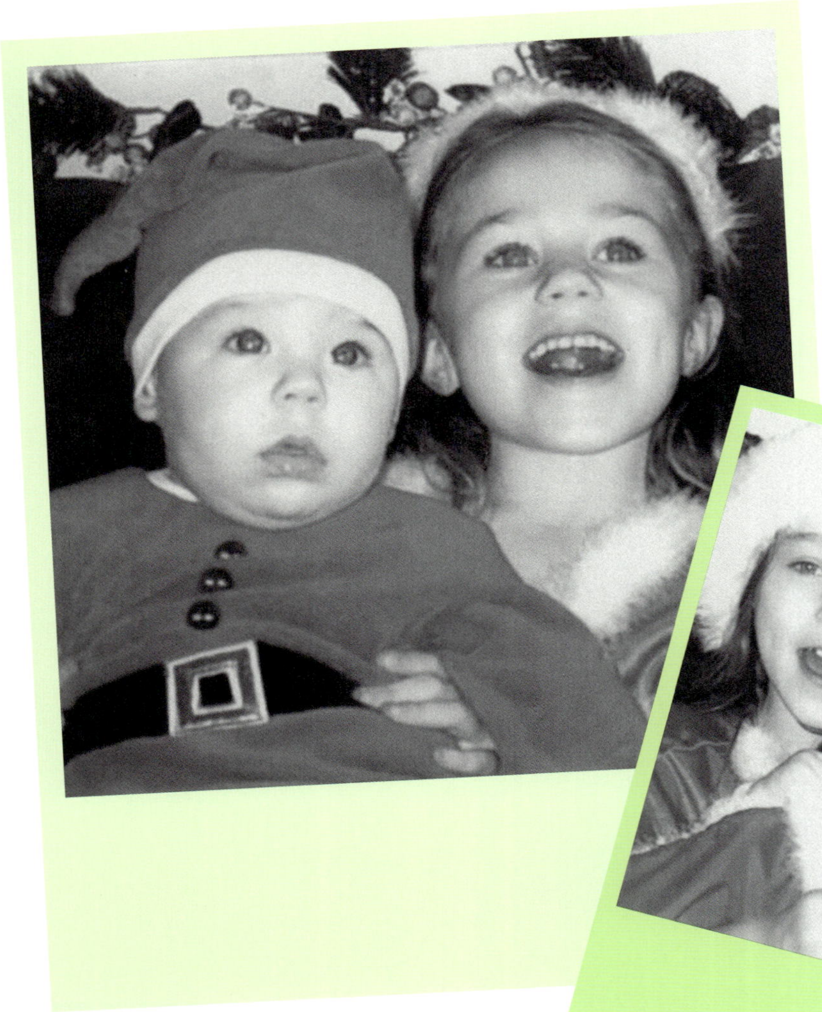

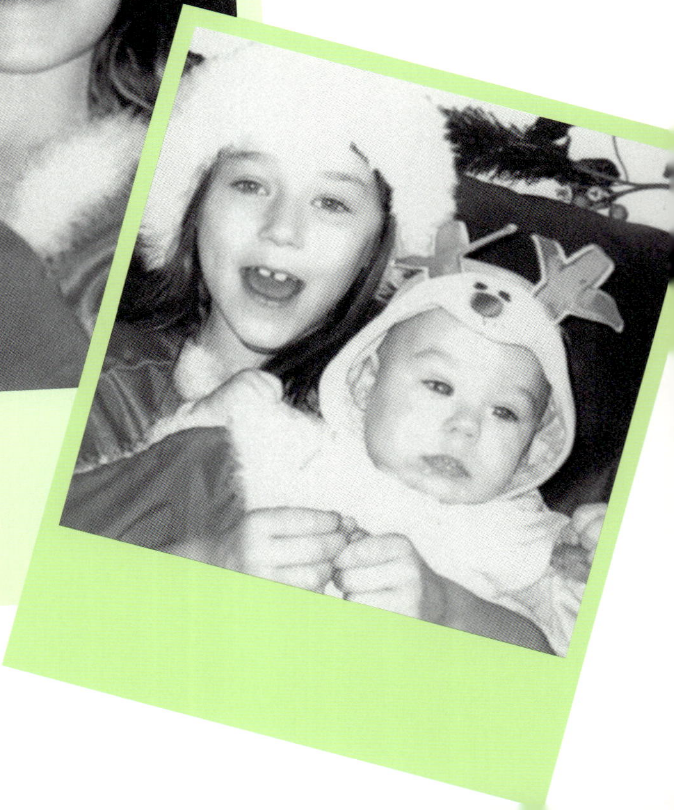

FIGURE 5: Urban Primary School Boys

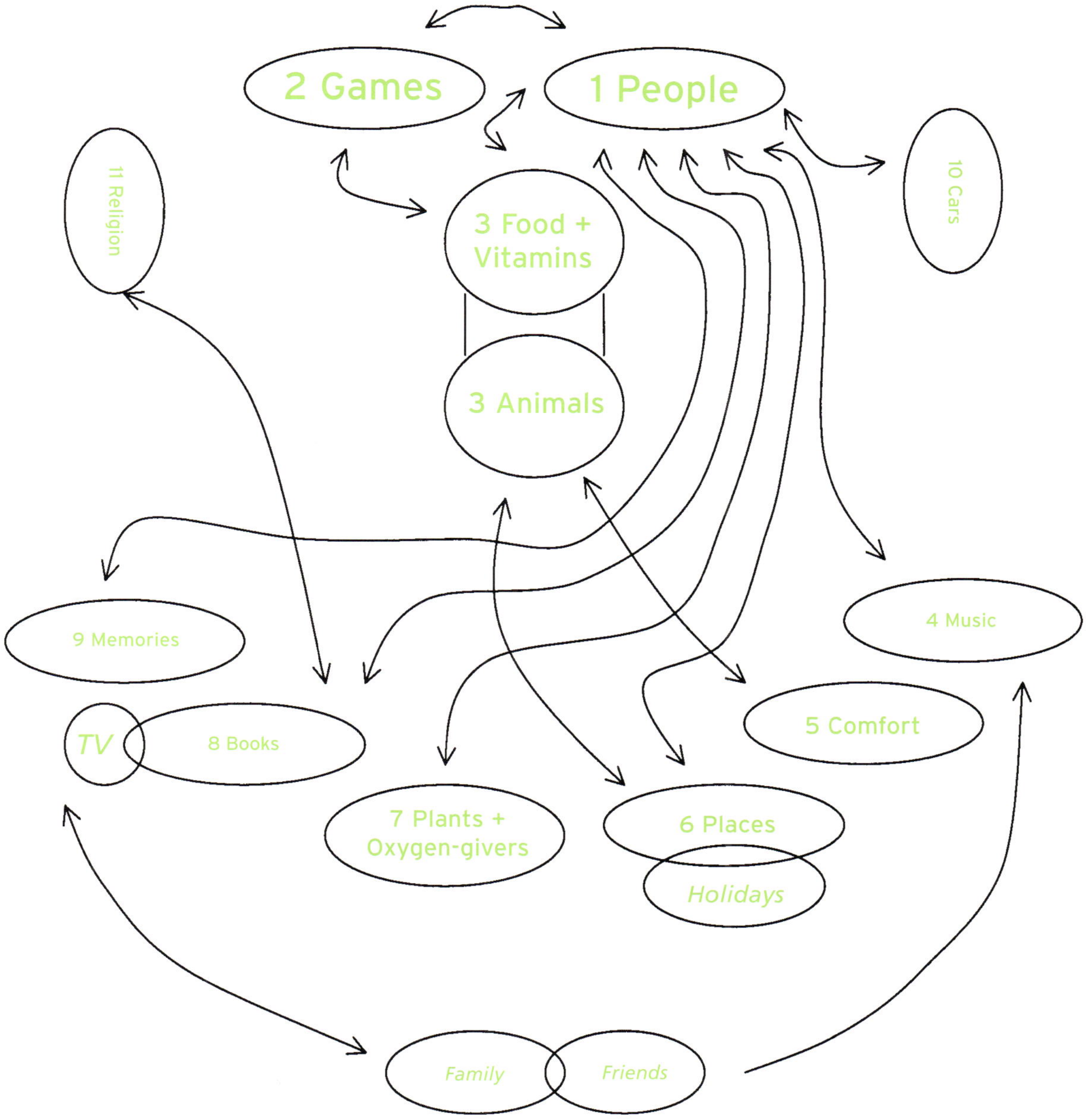

JOINT URBAN PRIMARY SCHOOL

A number of categories have been altered or subsumed into each other for this jointly constructed schema (Figure 6). 'Celebrations' comes from both the 'religious celebrations' and 'birthdays', although there was some heated discussion regarding whether birthdays were important for well-being. There was also intense discussion regarding the importance of 'religion', which does find its way into this joint schema albeit as the least important category. The new category 'transportation' includes both 'cars' and 'bikes'. 'TV' from the boys' schema has been added to the 'possessions' category from the girls' schema. 'Plants and oxygen-givers' from the boys' schema have been added into the 'environment' category from the girls' schema to make the category 'environment'. 'Comfort', originally from the boys' schema, and 'St. Valentine's Day' originally from the girls' schema, are both missing here. 'Medicine', the category that the girls had added to their schema, is also missing from the joint schema.

This schema should be read from left to right, with those on the left being most important for well-being and those on the right least important. Viewed vertically, it appears as an inverted question mark; however, it was reported that the intention was to represent a snake. Those categories that are touching each other on the schema were viewed as being intrinsically intertwined. In three of the sets of categories the categories are numbered, indicating order of importance. Thus in the first group, 'family' comes first, followed by 'friends' and then (other) 'people'. In the third group, 'pets/animals' comes first, followed jointly by 'playing' and 'games', and in the fourth group, 'comfort' and 'possessions' come joint first, followed by 'celebrations'. In all other groups, the categories were considered to be equal in importance. All children who were present during the construction of this schema signed the finished product, although for reasons of preserving their anonymity this is not represented in Figure 6.

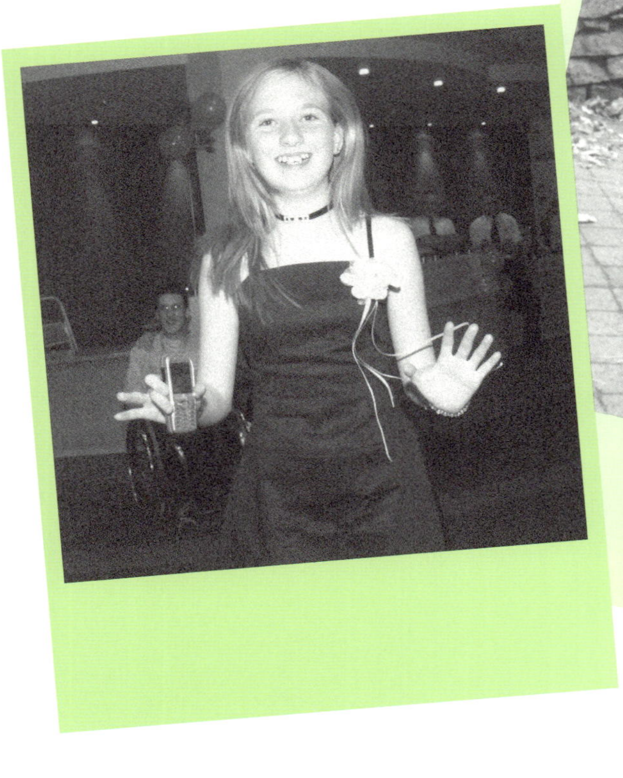

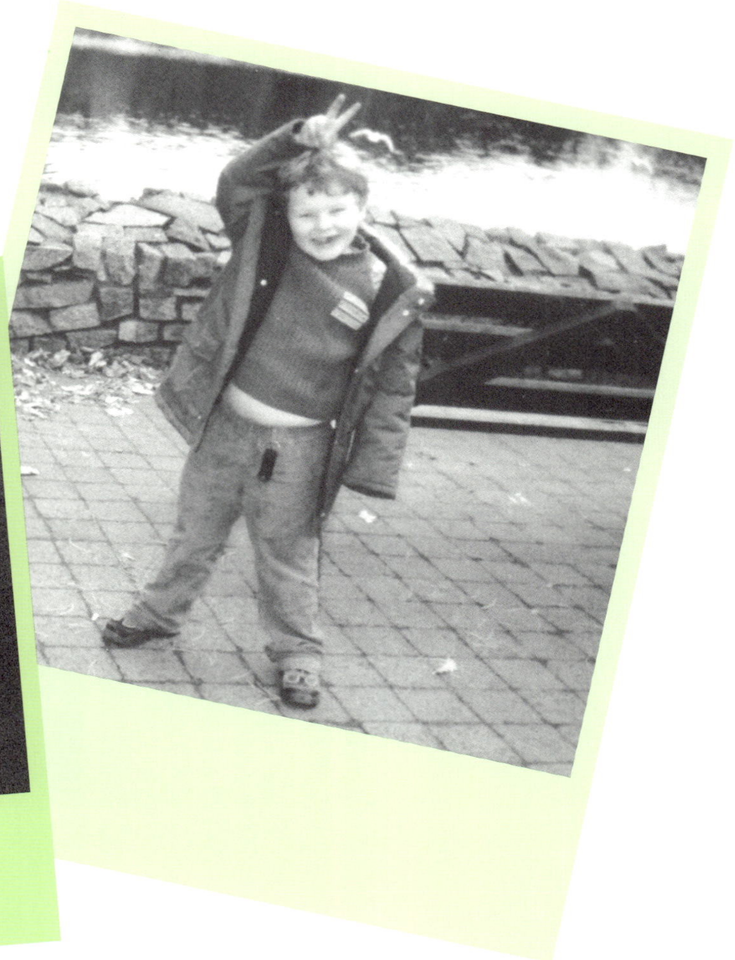

FIGURE 6: Joint Urban Primary School

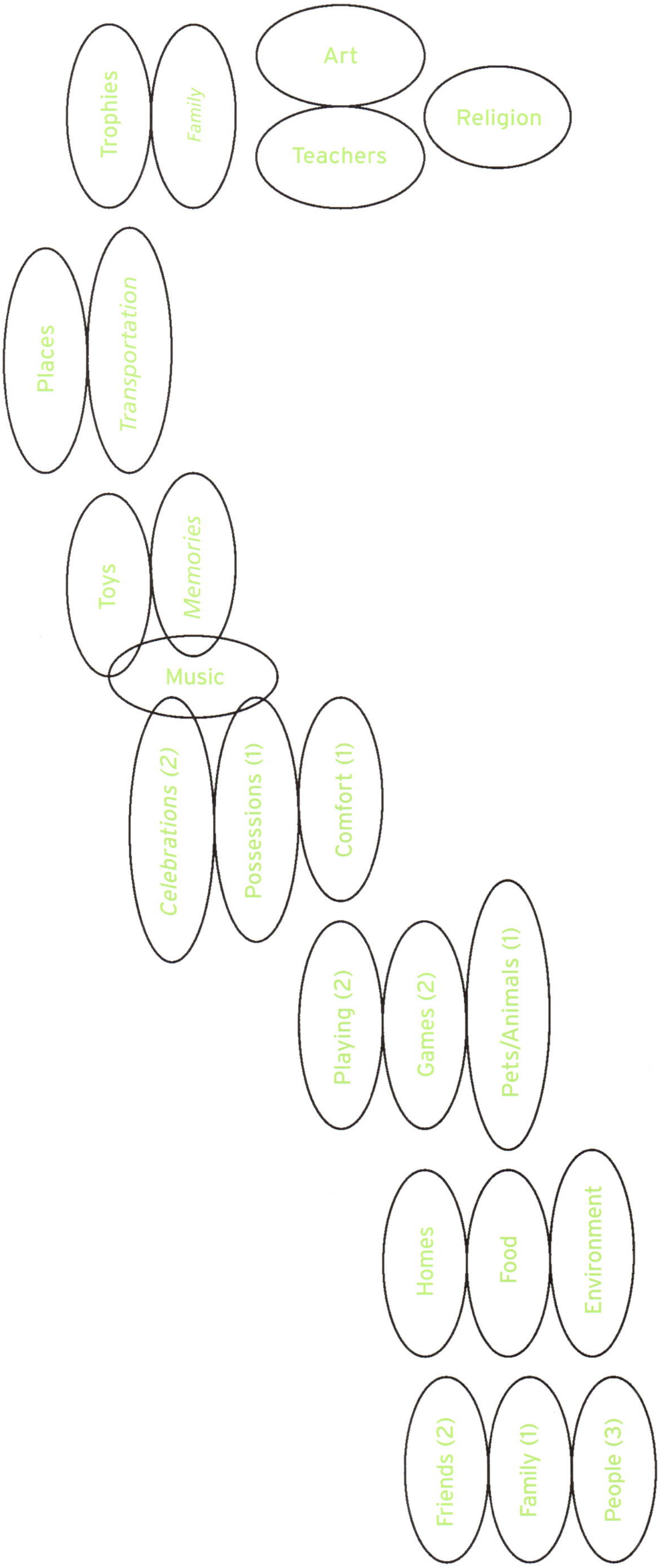

RURAL POST-PRIMARY SCHOOL GIRLS

The girls working on this schema development did not add new categories nor did they create new categories from combinations of the originals. However, they did merge categories. 'Pets' were merged with 'horses', 'favourite places' with 'bedrooms' and 'music', 'computers and playstations' with 'TV' and 'phones', 'magazines' with 'stuff' and 'teddies', 'bus/bus driver' with 'cars', and 'sports' with 'trophies and medals'. Thus they reduced the original 29 categories to 20.

This schema (Figure 7) should be read from top to bottom and left to right. Thus 'family' was considered most important for well-being, followed by 'friends', while 'Foróige club' followed by 'fags' (cigarettes) were the least important. None of the girls were members of Foróige, which may explain this placement. There was some dispute within the group about the relative importance of 'clothes' for well-being; however, it appears at number 4 here.

During the construction of this schema 'money' emerged as a factor of major importance. It was described as providing independence. These girls identified 'jobs' as a potential category that was missing, but elected not to include it. They described a job as a source of money and independence, *"giving you something to do"*. In addition they agreed that you *"appreciate something more if you have to work for it"*. This relationship between money and work is represented by the connection between 'money' and 'children/baby-sit' in the schema. With connections to 10 other categories, 'money' is the most connected category in this schema. It has connections to 'family', 'children/baby sit' (both sources of money), 'clothes', 'food', 'favourite places/bedrooms/beds/music', 'computers + playstations/TV/phones, pets/horses, bus/bus driver/cars', 'magazines/stuff/teddies, and fags'.

Another issue that arose during this session was the importance of role models, hence the connection between 'magazines/stuff/teddies' and 'teachers'. Magazines were described as providing information on people you look up to and 'teachers' were also people you looked up to. The girls pointed out that the category 'teachers' includes teachers outside the school setting, such as those who give grinds or teach music, dance and so on.

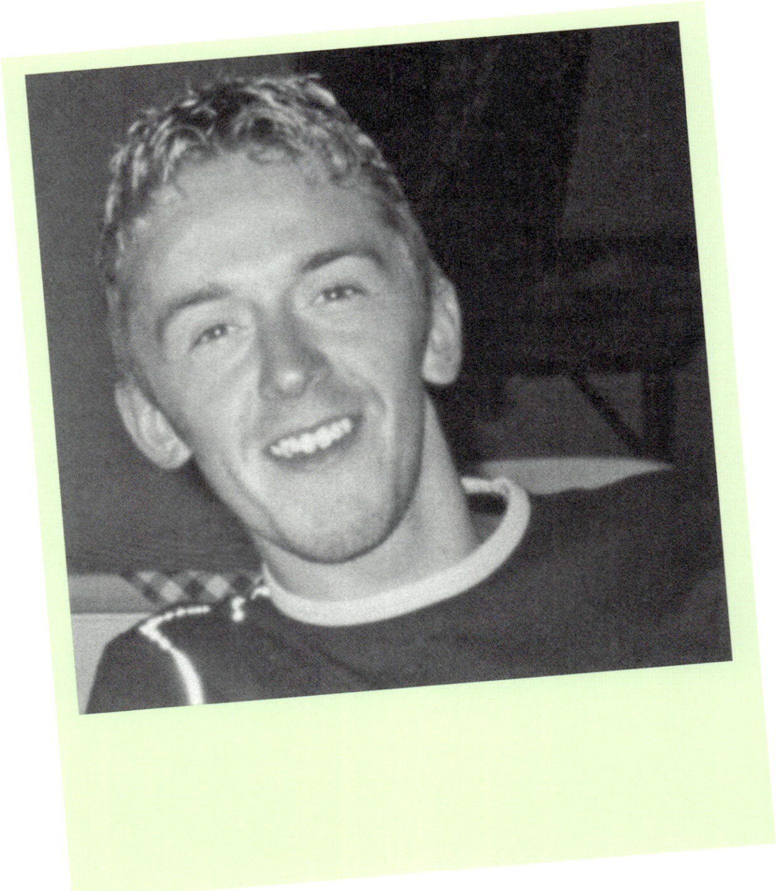

FIGURE 7: Rural Post-Primary School Girls

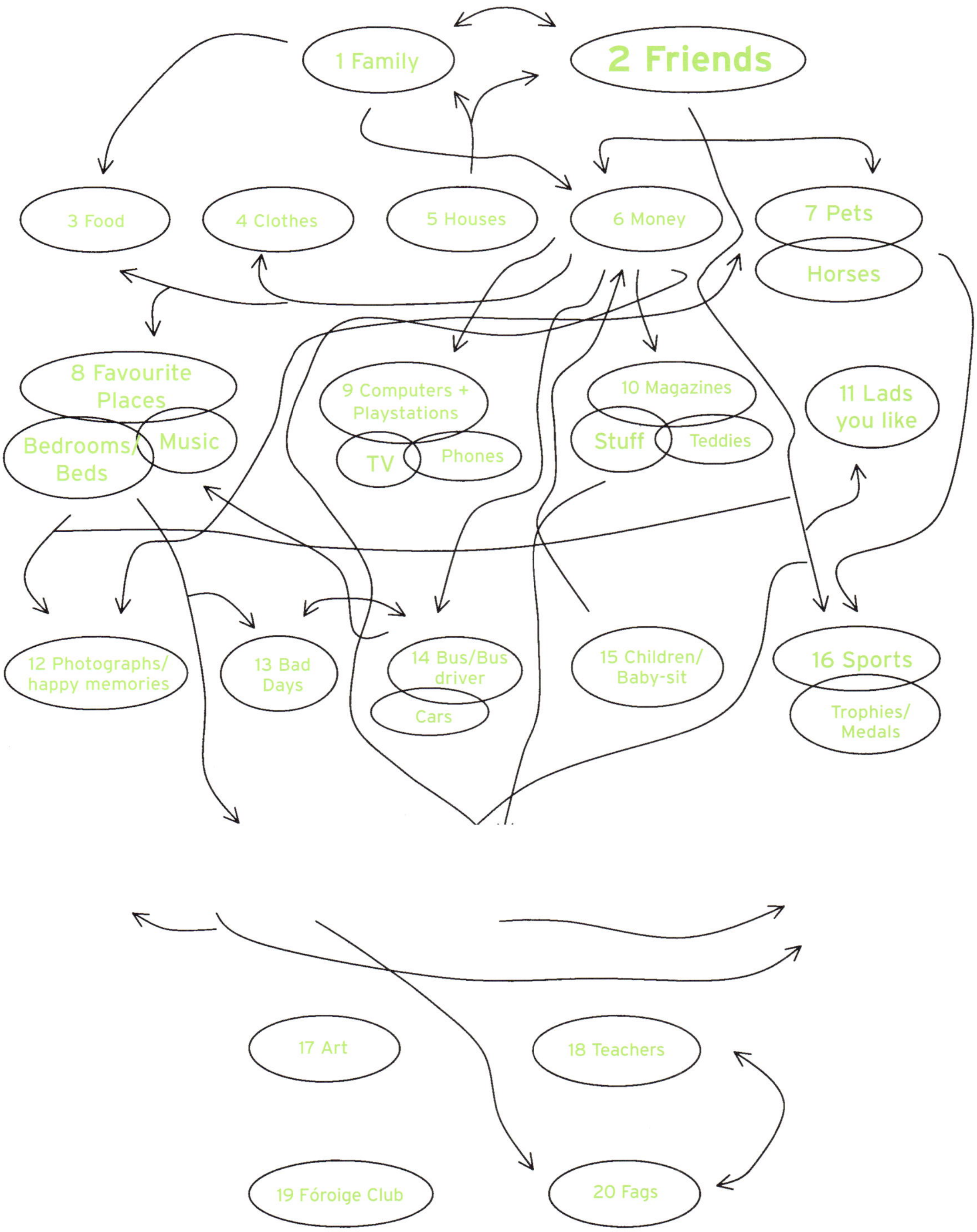

RURAL POST-PRIMARY SCHOOL BOYS

The boys who constructed this schema did not merge any of the original categories with each other nor did they group categories together. They did add four new categories: 'girls', 'celebrities e.g. Britney', 'movies' and 'gambling'. Most discussion took place regarding the category 'celebrities, e.g. Britney' since they argued that famous people were important role models for them. One of the boys insisted that the category 'gambling' was included because he felt that slot machines were a very important aspect of his own life.

Although the categories are not numbered, this schema (Figure 8) should be read as a flowchart (so described by the boys), reading from left to right on each line. Thus the most important category for well-being is the 'family', followed by 'friends' and 'girls', and the least important categories are 'sheep' and 'sheds'. The boys pointed out that all categories in the first line were necessary for well-being. The boys discussed the relative importance of education, which can help you to get a good job and make money. There was some disagreement as to the importance of 'school' for this purpose, which explains 'money' being placed on the first line and 'school' on the second. This is the only gender-specific schema that does not include connections representing relationships between categories. These boys said that all the categories were connected to each other.

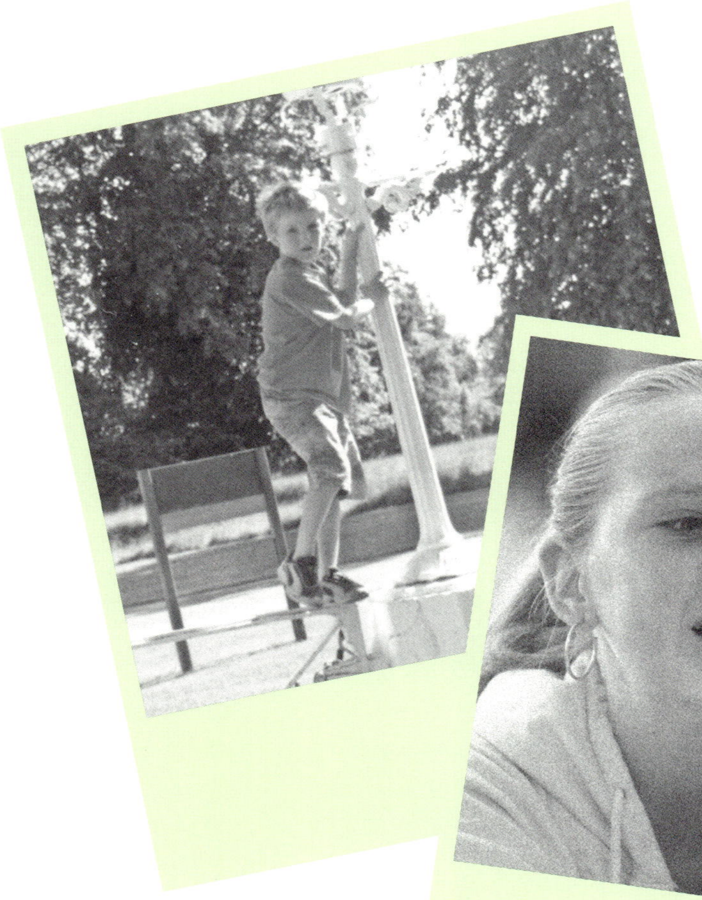

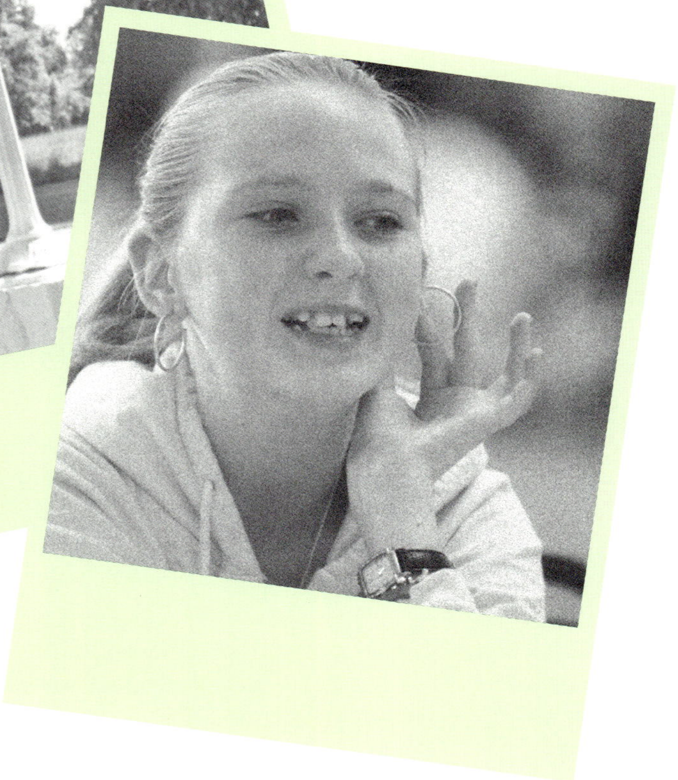

FIGURE 8: Rural Post-Primary School Boys

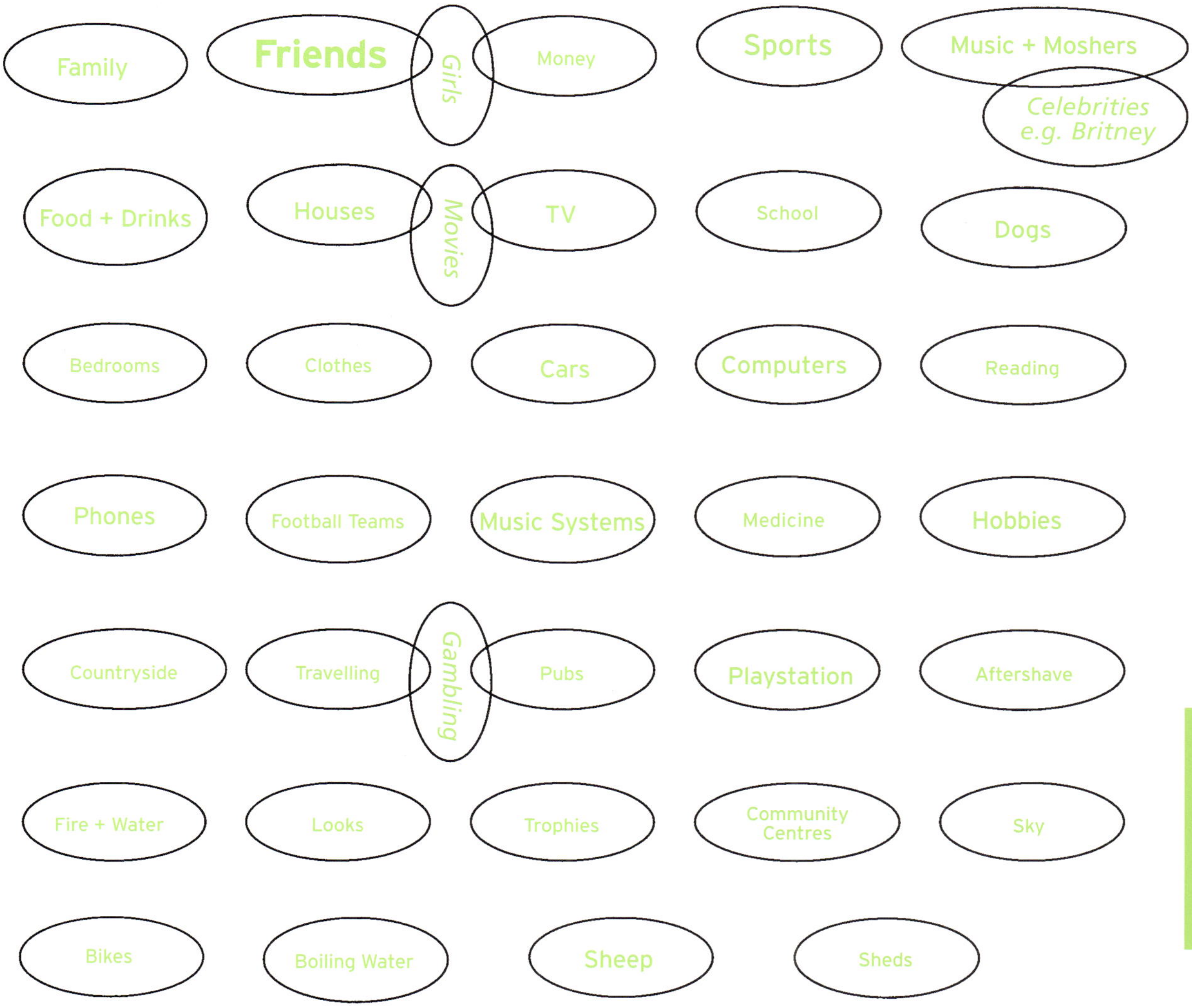

JOINT RURAL POST-PRIMARY SCHOOL

This joint schema includes two new categories: 'socialising' (including pubs and clubs) and 'opposite sex', comprised of 'guys you like' from the girls' schema and 'girls' from the boys' schema. A number of categories from both the single sex schemata were not brought forward to this one. 'Moshers', 'gambling', 'boiling water', 'sheep' and 'sheds' from the boys' schema and 'bus/bus driver' and 'foróige club' from the girls' schema are missing here. 'Money', ranked 6th out of 20 by the girls (and the most connected category) and 4th out of 38 by the boys, is also not included here. The joint group placed a number of the categories together. The overlapping oval shapes and a single number for each group represent this. The extent of the renegotiation required to construct joint schema is evident here, particularly in the comparison between the original schema and the jointly constructed schema. For example, categories 8 and 9 from the girls' schema ('favourite places/bedrooms/beds/music and computers' and 'playstation/TV/phones') have been deconstructed and placed at different levels of the hierarchy within the joint schema.

This schema (Figure 9) should be read in the same way as the post-primary rural girls' schema, from top left to bottom right, with the categories numbered in order of their importance for well-being. Thus the most important category is 'family' followed by 'friends' and the least is 'bad days'.

During the discussion that took place when this schema was being constructed, a number of important issues arose. These included the importance of school and education; thus 'school' and 'teachers' are placed 10th here, which is up from 'school' at 12th in the boys' schema and 'teachers' at 18th in the girls' schema. This group also discussed the relative importance of 'looks', 'celebrities' and 'TV'. Both boys and girls described 'celebrities' as people you can look up to, while the boys particularly stressed the importance of television for keeping you happy, occupied and informed. The group agreed that it was difficult to construct a hierarchy (though this is what they themselves decided to do) because everything is important.

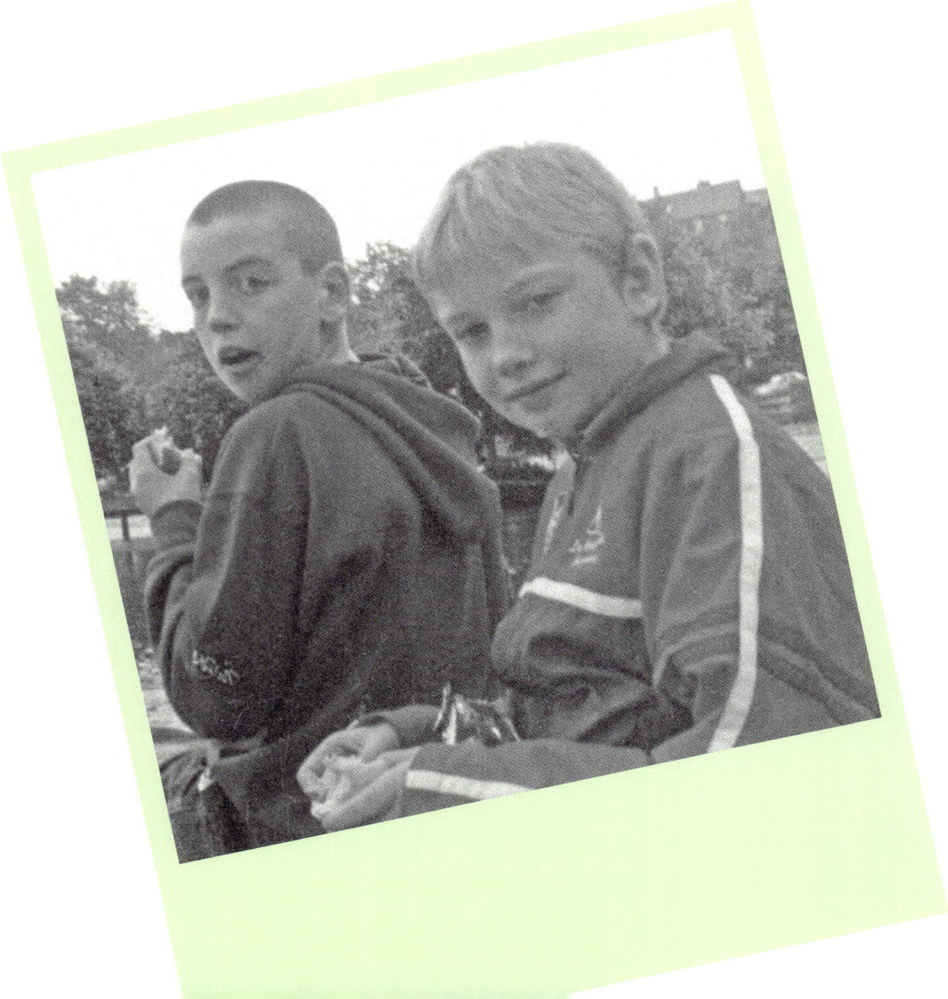

FIGURE 9: Joint Rural Post-Primary School

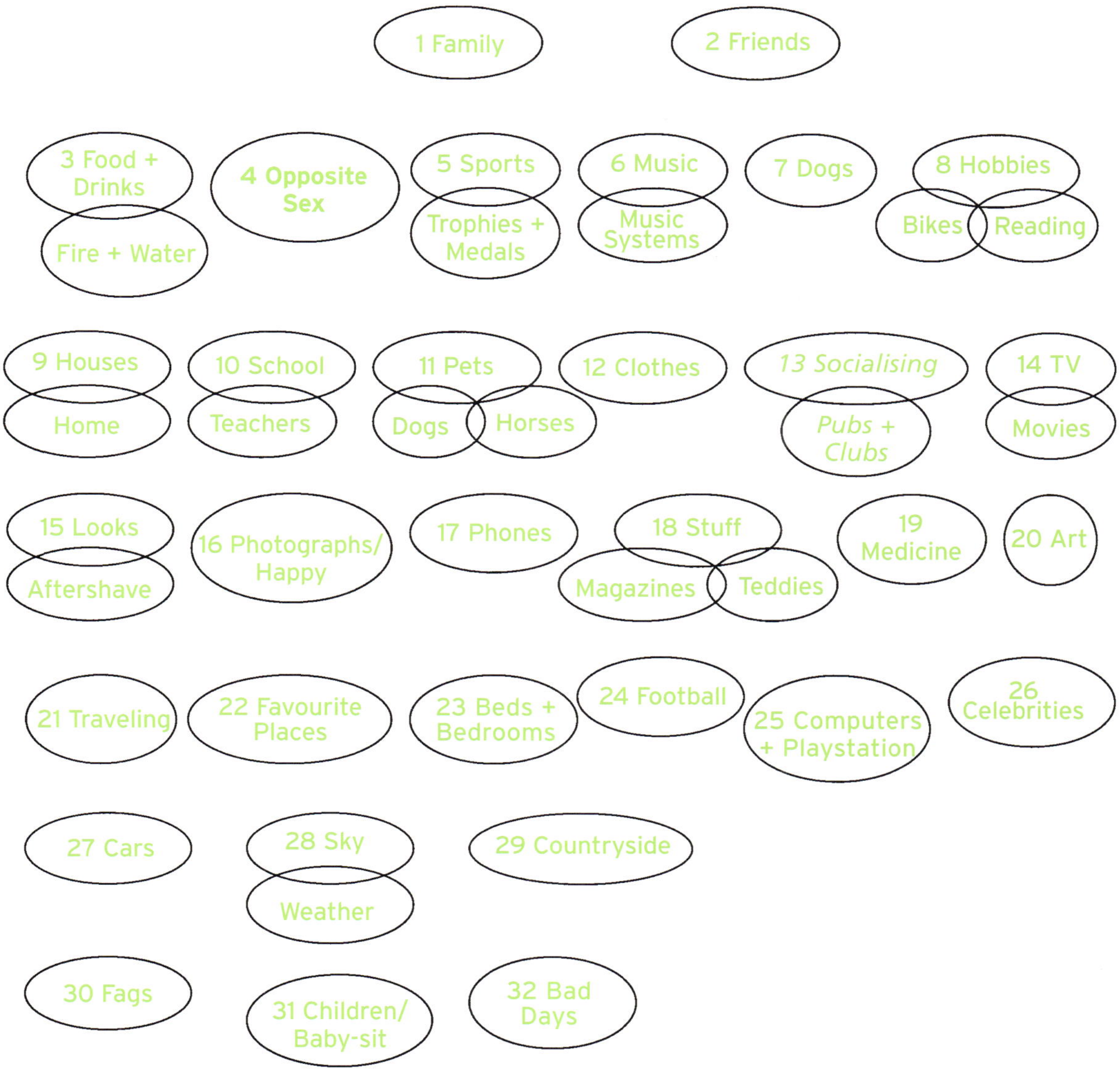

URBAN POST-PRIMARY SCHOOL GIRLS

A number of the original categories are merged in this schema (Figure 10), all labeled in bold:

- 'outside' - comprised of 'outside', 'houses' and 'streets and cars'
- 'culture' - comprised of 'culture' and 'art work'
- 'friends' - comprised of 'best friends' and 'school friends'
- 'hobbies' - comprised of 'hobbies' and 'music'
- 'entertainment' - comprised of 'books' and 'entertainment'
- 'me' - comprised of 'cranky', 'pj's + bedrooms', 'special occasions', 'memories', 'shoes/clothes', 'stuff' (make-up, phones, magazines, etc.)

There is also a new category, that of 'school' (which is italicised). These girls argued that school was important for well-being because *"education is very important"*.

'Friends' are connected with 11 other categories, which is only eclipsed by the category 'me'. Although not written on the physical schema completed by the girls, it was agreed that 'me' was connected with all 17 other categories, and the researchers agreed to ensure that this was appropriately represented. This schema is extremely complex as recognised by the girls involved in its construction. The girls refused to add any more connections because it was getting *"too messy"*. They had wanted to connect 'school' with 'friends' and 'food' with 'family', but didn't want to *"mess up"* the depiction of the schema any further.

There was considerable discussion regarding the category 'me'. Girls argued that if you *"didn't look after yourself, what's the point, no-one else will"*. None of the girls involved in the schema development had a pet and none of them were involved in charities, therefore both of these categories were ranked relatively low in importance. Along with the category 'me', the category 'outside' became a focus of group discussion. The girls reported that it was important to get out of their houses *"because you need your freedom"*. They also emphasised the relative importance of guys and children *"because going to be with them and have children, so more important than friends as friends won't feature in a few years"*.

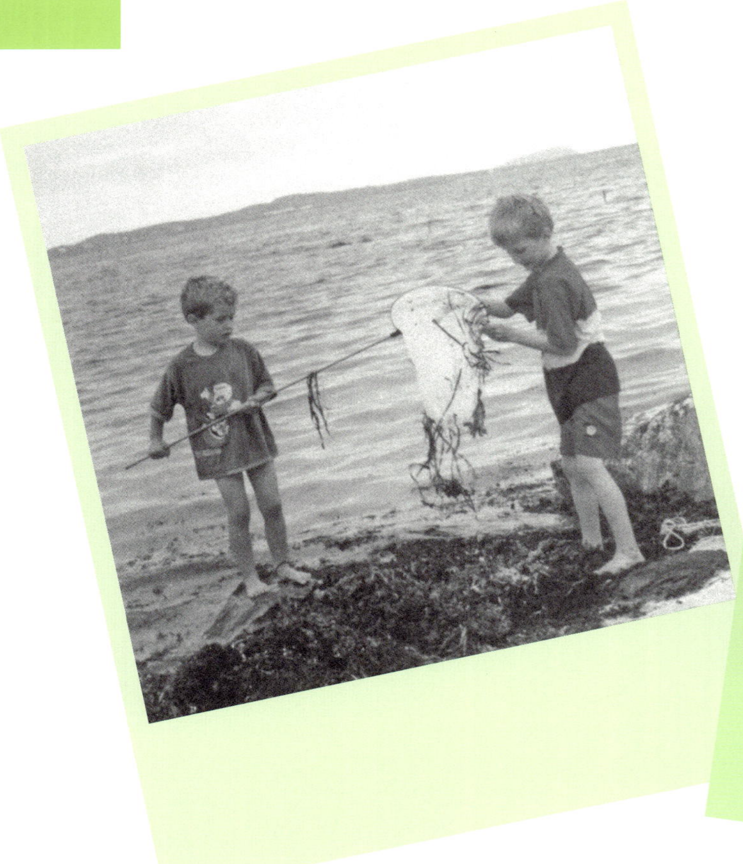

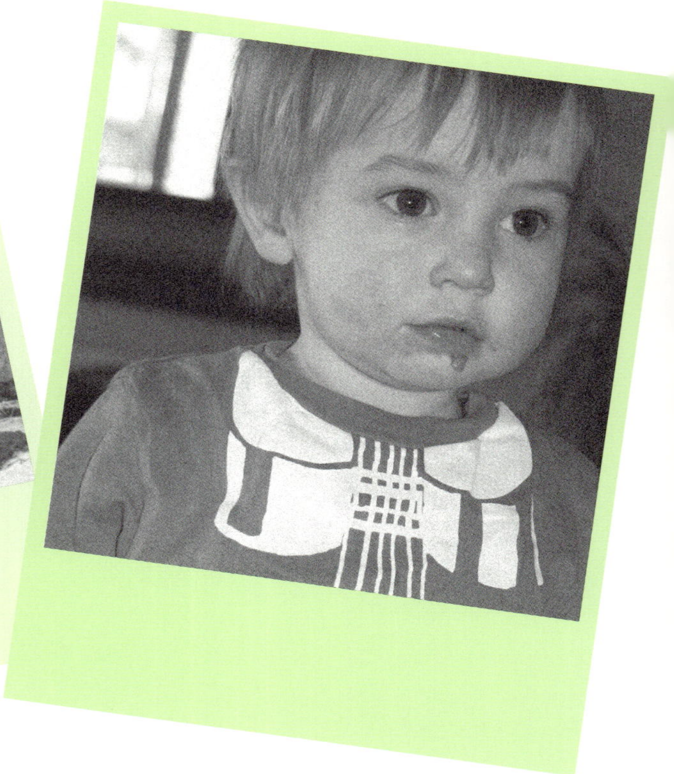

FIGURE 10: Urban Post-Primary School Girls

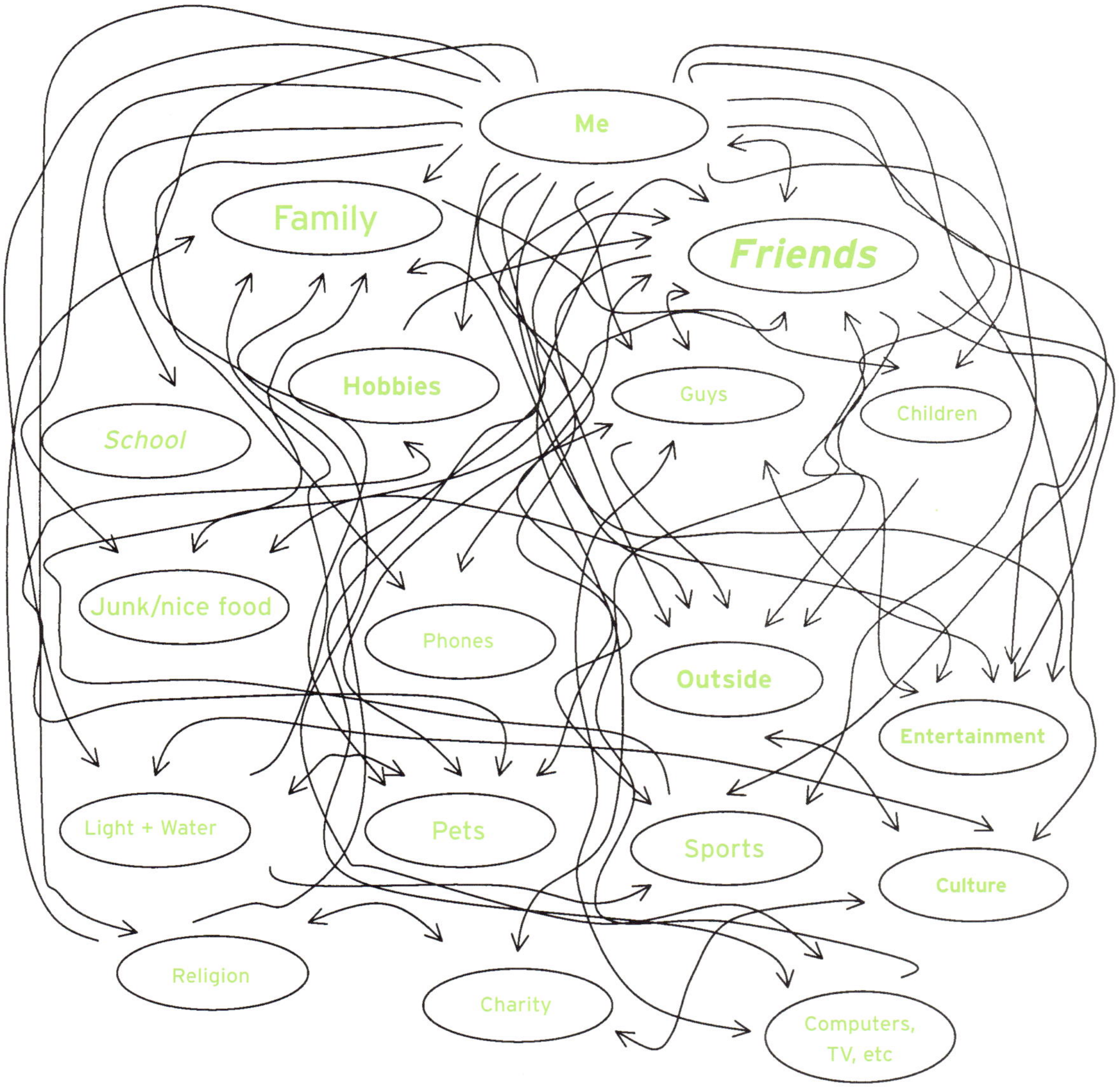

URBAN POST-PRIMARY SCHOOL BOYS

The schema in Figure 11 is characterised by a spiral, starting with number 1 ('family'), moving diagonally from left to right and then up to the top right-hand corner and around the edges of the schema anti-clockwise until number 20 ('books'), then diagonally to the upper left, ending with number 21 ('miscellaneous'). The direction is indicated by the solid arrows. Number 1 ('family') was considered most important, with increasing numbers indicating a decrease in importance. All categories from the original classification were employed.

Two specific categories are very well connected, that of 'friends' (connected to 'gardens', 'places', 'sexy photos', 'school', 'playing sport', 'rooms', 'mobile phones') and that of 'rooms' (connected to 'friends', 'food', 'sexy photos', 'music', 'books', 'technology', 'miscellaneous'). 'Watching/following sports' and 'travel' were both unconnected.

In this context, the category 'rooms' was conceptualised as bedrooms and the boys involved in the schema development discussed the centrality of their rooms to their lives. Their bedrooms were described as the central location for personal and social activity. This contrasts strongly with the urban post-primary school girls, who identified the category 'outside' (meaning outside the home, on the streets) as the key location for their lives. The boys commented negatively on the importance of school for well-being. However, while placing it on the schema they noted that in school they learn things, make friends and play sports, and also that they *"hang out with the lads from school outside school"*.

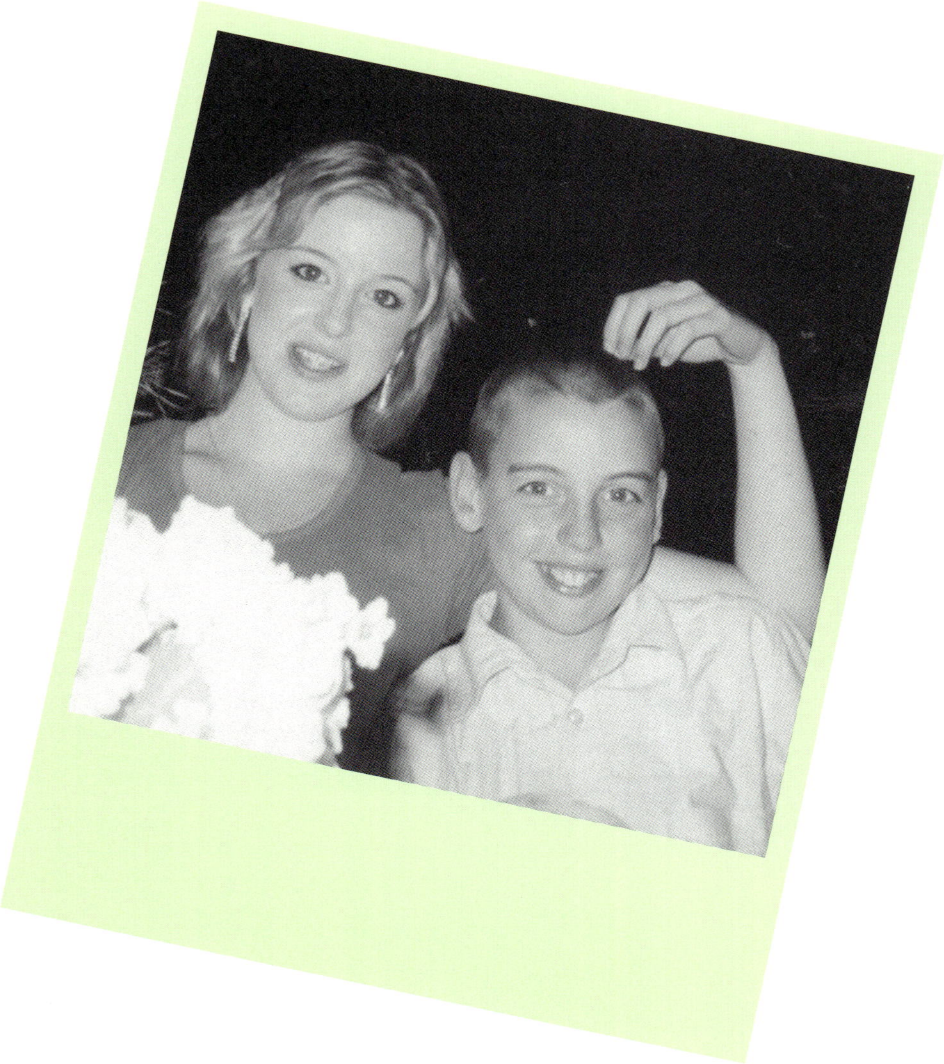

FIGURE 11: Urban Post-Primary School Boys

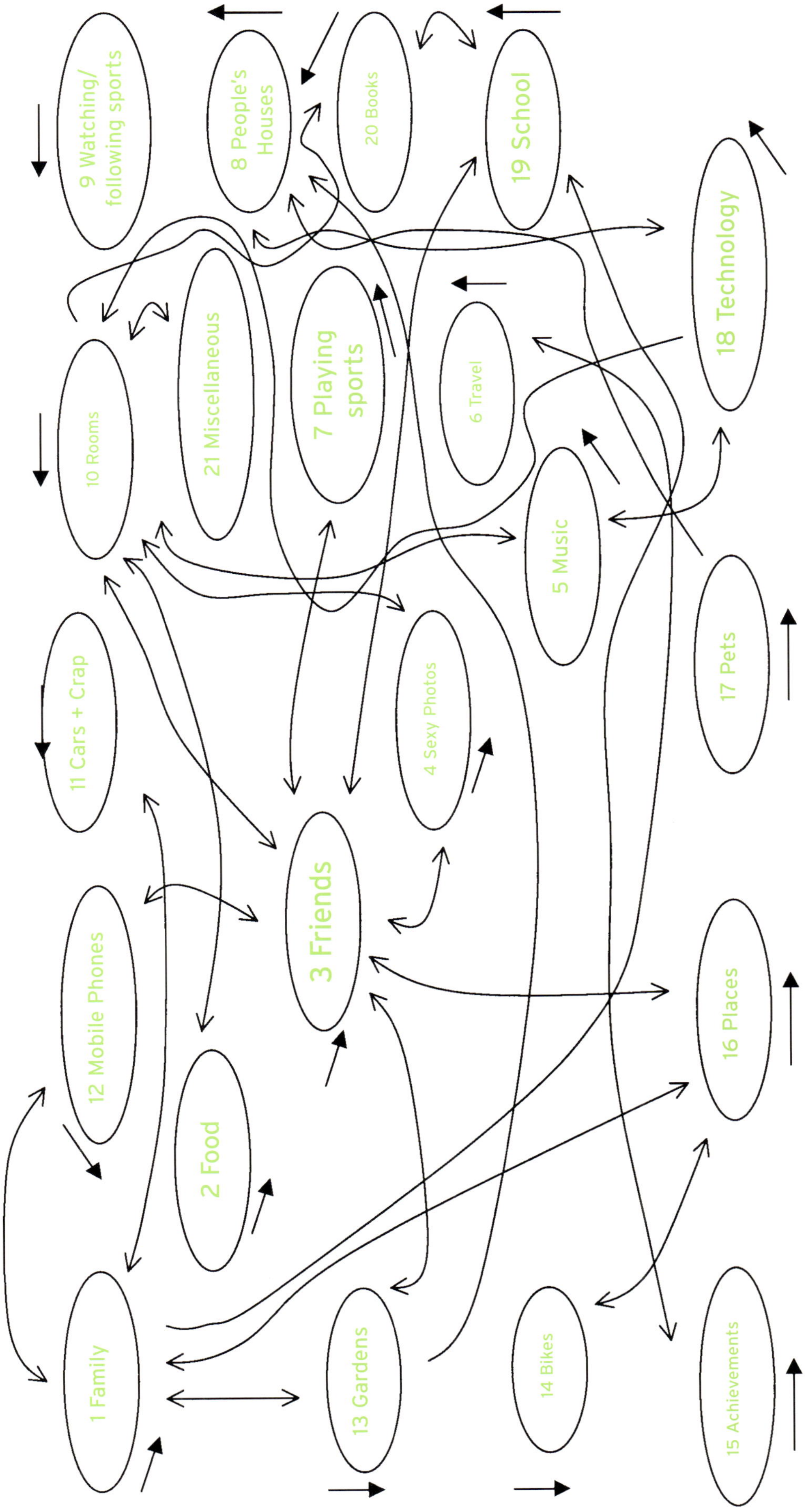

JOINT URBAN POST-PRIMARY SCHOOL

This joint schema includes most of the categories included from both the girls' and boys' original schema and the category of 'sleep' was added during the session, 'technology' from the boys' original schema is included in the category 'computers, TV, etc.', but both 'places' and 'watching/following sport' are missing from the joint schema. No categories are missing from the original girls' schema. A number of sets of categories were placed together and this is illustrated by overlapping categories in the schema. 'School', 'books', 'achievements' and 'art' were all considered to be aspects of 'schools', while 'rooms' and 'hobbies' were seen to include the categories 'computers, TV, etc.' and 'miscellaneous. 'Religion' was placed with 'charity'. The category 'best friends' is brought forward here from the girls' schema. It had been merged with 'school friends' to form 'friends' in the girls' schema, but appears here in its own right.

In this schema (Figure 12), as with the girls' schema, the category 'me' was placed at the centre of the pattern and the other categories were placed a distance from it. However, this did not continue throughout the whole process of joint schema development because the children got frustrated constantly moving the categories around. The categories are numbered as to their importance for well-being, and this process involved considerable debate. Gender differences emerged: with the exception of one boy, the boys were not interested in 'school', but did consider their 'bedrooms' to be very important to their well-being. On the other hand, girls argued that 'school' was important for their future, but were more interested in 'outside' as a location within which to live their lives. The girls were not enthusiastic about 'computers and TV' or 'music' being considered important for well-being. The category 'me', originally from the girls' schema, had been created from an amalgamation of a number of categories, including 'stuff'. When 'me' was brought forward to the joint schema, the significance of 'stuff' within it was lost. However, given that the boys brought forward the category 'shoes and clothes', the girls argued that this *"was like stuff"* and thus that concept was re-introduced here.

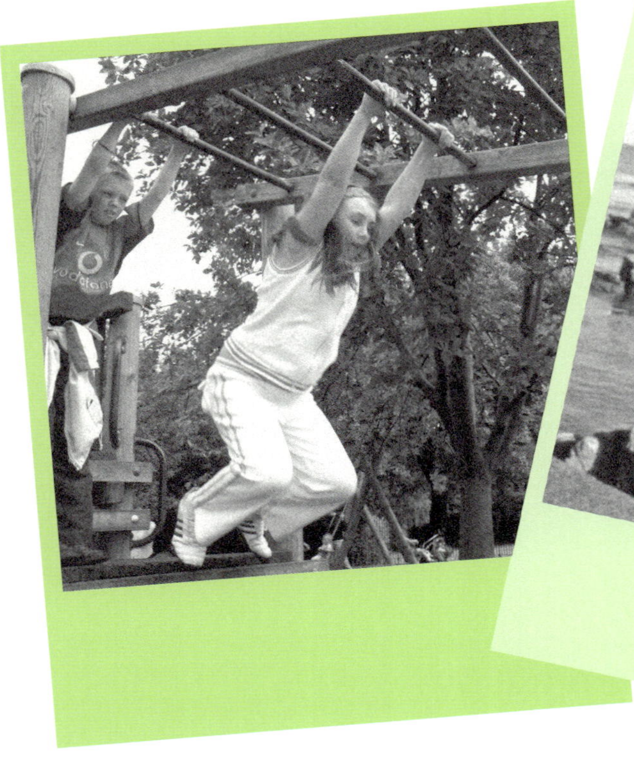

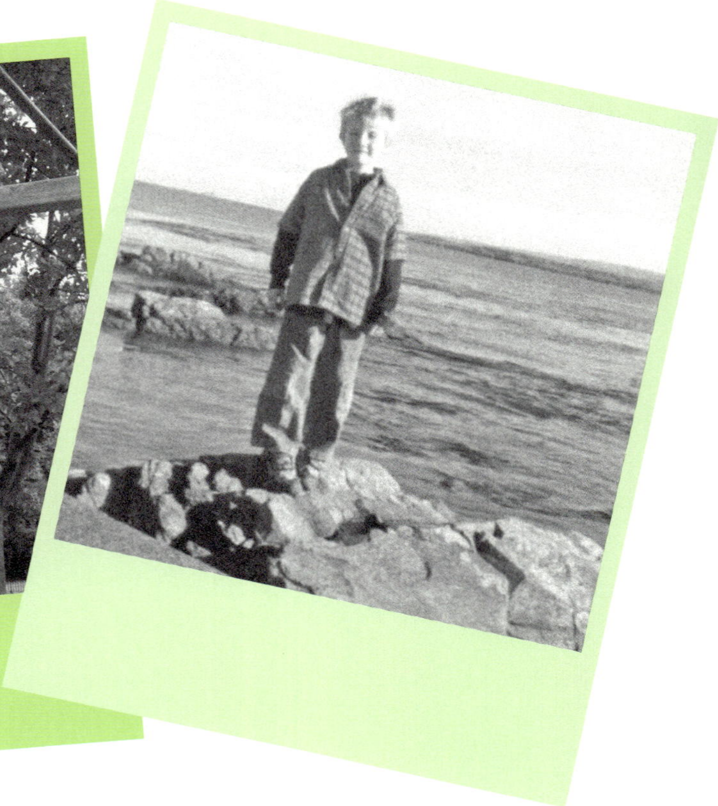

FIGURE 12: Joint Urban Post-Primary School

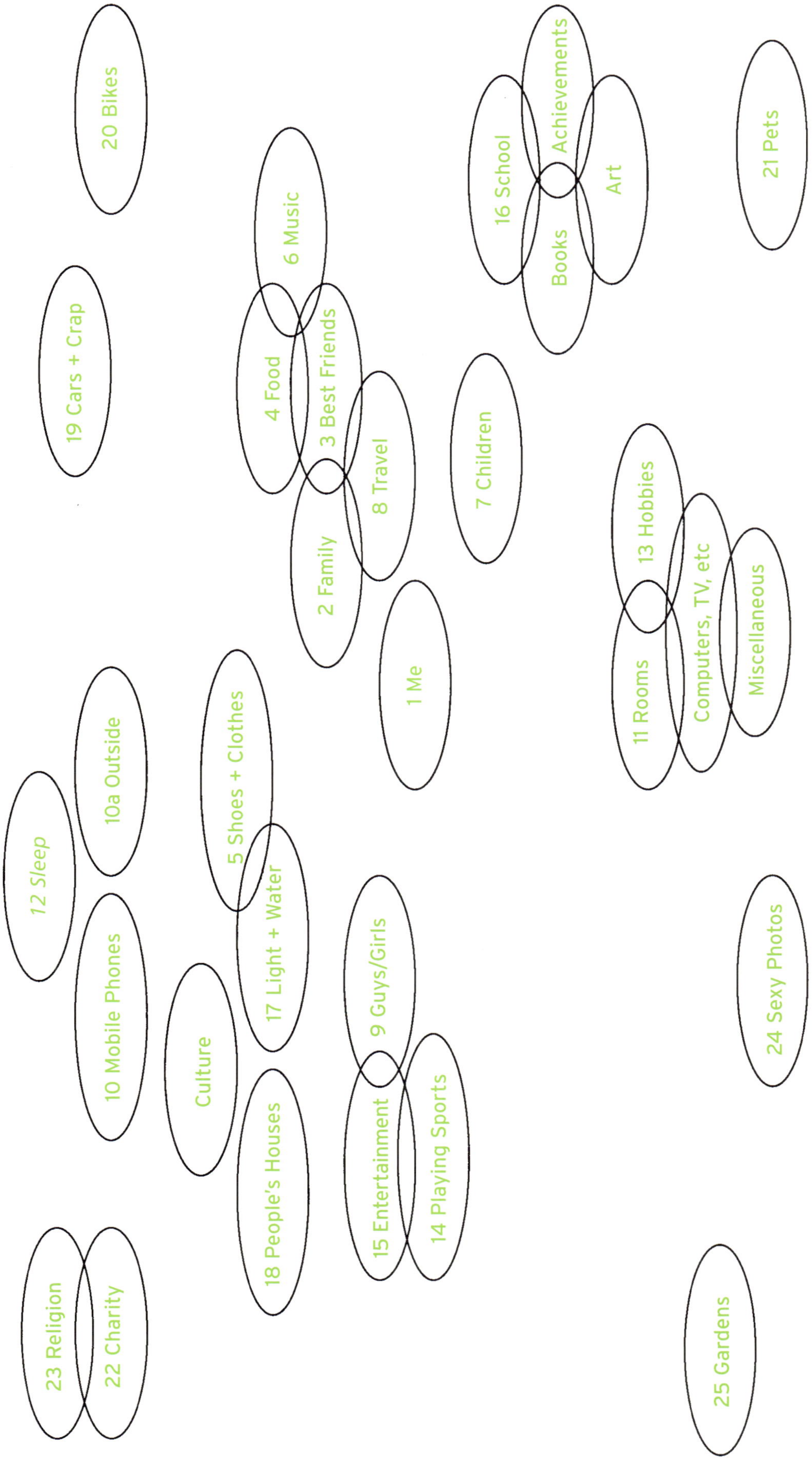

57

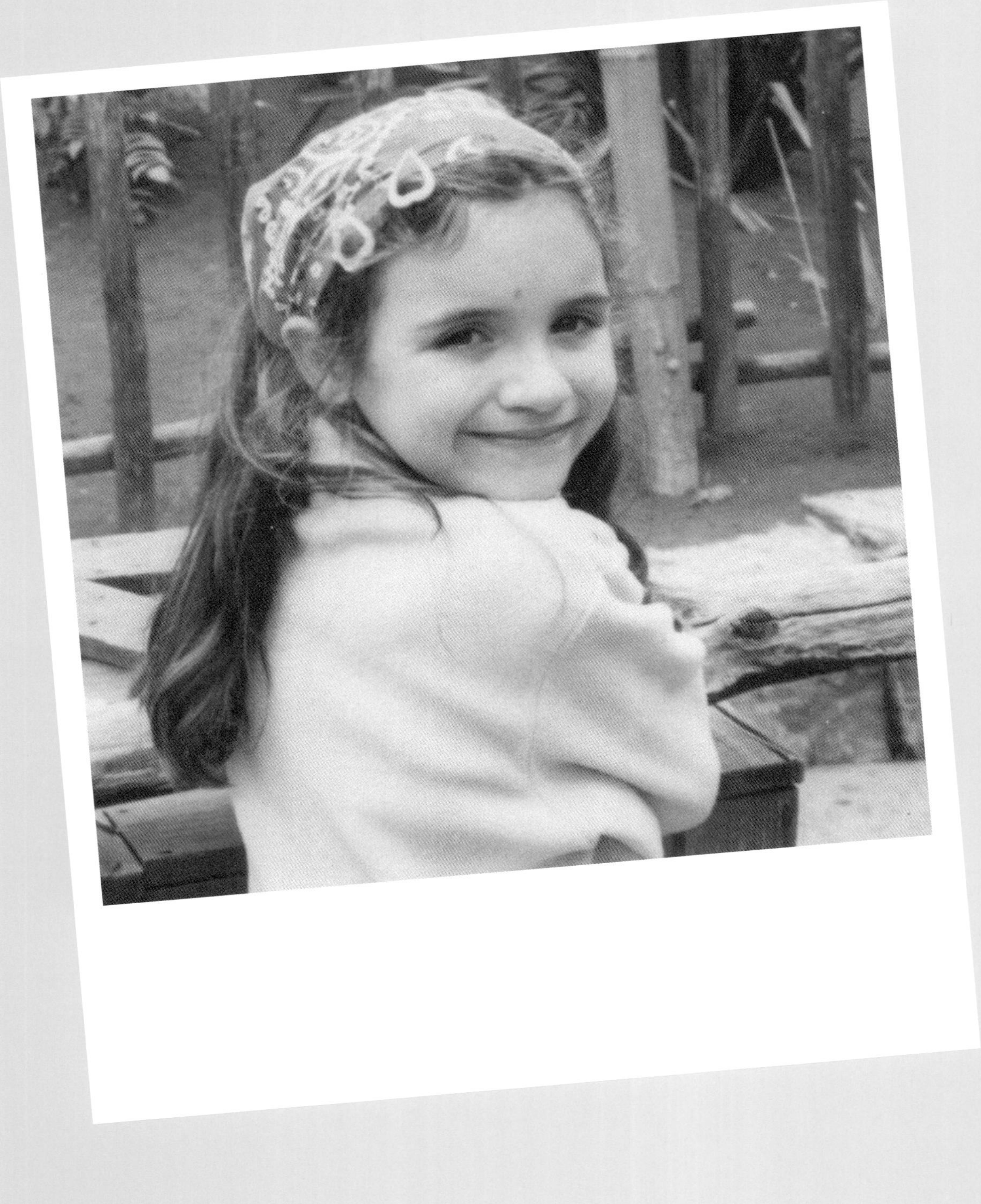

PHASE 4: FINAL INTEGRATION OF SCHEMATA

The final integration of the developed schemata took place in a youth café/centre in a regional town. This location was neither rural nor urban, but had aspects of both. The group that were invited to participate were the youth advisory committee (i.e. the group workroom involved in an advisory capacity with the running of the centre). This group knew each other well and had worked together in the past on building group trust, cohesion and decision-making. The session with this group was scheduled to take place out of school hours in a group workroom within the youth centre. This session commenced as the other group sessions, with introductions, setting ground rules and introducing the concept of well-being. The young people were given copies of the gender-specific schemata (n=8) as developed by the children involved in phase 3. They were given some time to look at the schemata and to ask questions about them. Then they were broken into three mixed gender groups.

The first group was to identify similarities and differences across gender, the second across age groups and the third across urban/rural children. They wrote their responses on flipcharts. The primary objective of this exercise was to facilitate the groups' understanding of the content and patterns in the developed schemata. This work is represented in Table 16. The lists in this table are as provided by the children during the final data integration session in the youth centre. There are some overlaps in the differences and similarities columns identified by the children (particularly in the urban/rural comparisons). The first column presents the similarity among girls and the second comprises the categories upon which girls do not all agree. The second set of columns present this same information for boys.

Next, the groups were brought together to work on the development of a schema of well-being that would represent - *all children* - boys, girls, urban, rural, primary and post-primary. The young people used coloured flashcards and developed their own category names to do this. The flashcards were organised and secured onto sheets of coloured A1 card. This session was also audio-recorded and the researchers took notes and were debriefed. These data are employed here to assist in the interpretation of the young people's work.

TABLE 16: Identified similarities and differences between schemata

GIRLS		BOYS		PRIMARY		POST-PRIMARY		URBAN/RURAL	
Similarities	*Differences*	*Similarities*	*Differences*	*Similarities*	*Differences*	*Similarities*	*Differences*	*Similarities*	*Differences*
Family	Themselves	Family	Girls	Friends	Holidays	Family	Food	Friends	Clothes
Friends	Teddies	Friends	Fun	Family	People	Friends	Me	Family	Children
Pets	Guys/girls	Cars	Memories	Video games + TV[1]	Sports+trophies	Music	Travel	Pets	Money
Religious Education	Flowers	Sports	Travel	Cars[2]	School (rural)	Guys/girls	Hobbies	Food	Houses
Food	Trophies	School	Pets	Pets/animals	Art	Money	Horses	Houses	School
Houses/homes	Children	Video games	Fishing	Places	Music	Sports	Stuff	Places	Teams
School/teachers	Money	TV	Community centre	Plants + Environment[3]	Memories	School	Light and water	Toys	Neighbours
Hobbies	Possessions	Reading	Sheep	Religion[4]	Comfort	Houses	Outside	Sport	Possessions
	Playing toys		Boiling water	Food	Clocks	Phones	Children	Music	Things to do
	Phones		Phones	Toys + playing[5]	Trampoline	TV	Charity	School	Travel
	Fags			Houses + rooms[6]	Fishing		Religion	Bikes	Books
	Clothes			Books and reading[7]	Laughing		Culture	Games	Sexy photos
	Environment				Energy + strength			Plants	Laughing
	Medicine				Teachers				Trampoline
	Entertainment				Neighbours				Memories
	Art				Things to do				Food
	Computers/ playstation				Possessions				
					Medicine				
					Birthday				
					Religious Celebrations				
					St. Valentine's Day				

[1]boys
[2]not urban girls
[3]not rural boys
[4]not rural boys
[5]not urban boys
[6]rural
[7]rural

The schema shown in Figure 13 was designed to represent the perspectives of all the groups of children involved in this research. All the 22 categories within it were chosen by the participants to correspond to those developed by other children. The children also chose the colours upon which to write the categories*; however, the colours themselves were not of significance beyond the rainbow effect that the group decided to employ. The category at the top of the outer rainbow 'family' was judged to be the most important, while 'friends' and 'food' were joint second, 'school' and 'houses' joint third, and so on.

The same applies to the lower rainbow, where 'cars' are most important. However the youth group was not as emphatic about the hierarchy in the second rainbow. The lower rainbow was deliberately placed just above the final categories of the outer rainbow, as the young people involved in its construction argued that all of the categories in the lower rainbow were more important than 'books + reading' or 'religion'.

Given that this schema was constructed to be representative of all children, it does not faithfully relate to the discussion that took place during its construction regarding the opinions of these young people about the factors which are important for their own well-being. For example, one of the boys reported that the main source of his own well-being was playing music; however he thought that this was not common among rural youth and so could not be too prominent within the hierarchy.

The young people involved in this final integration were asked what was missing from the schema as presented. One of the agreed gaps was happiness; they reported that being happy was the main thing that made and kept you well. In general, these young people emphasised the emotional aspects of the various categories.

** As this publication is in two-colour, it is not possible to reproduce the original colours selected by the children, in Figure 13.*

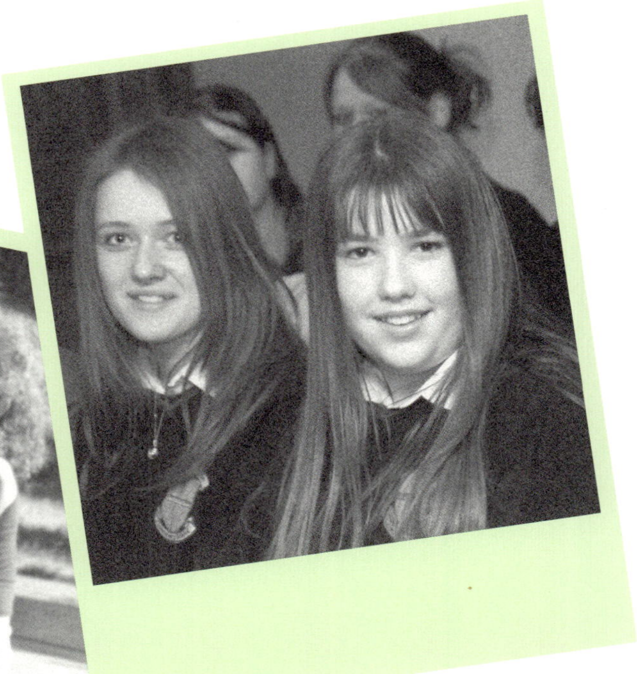

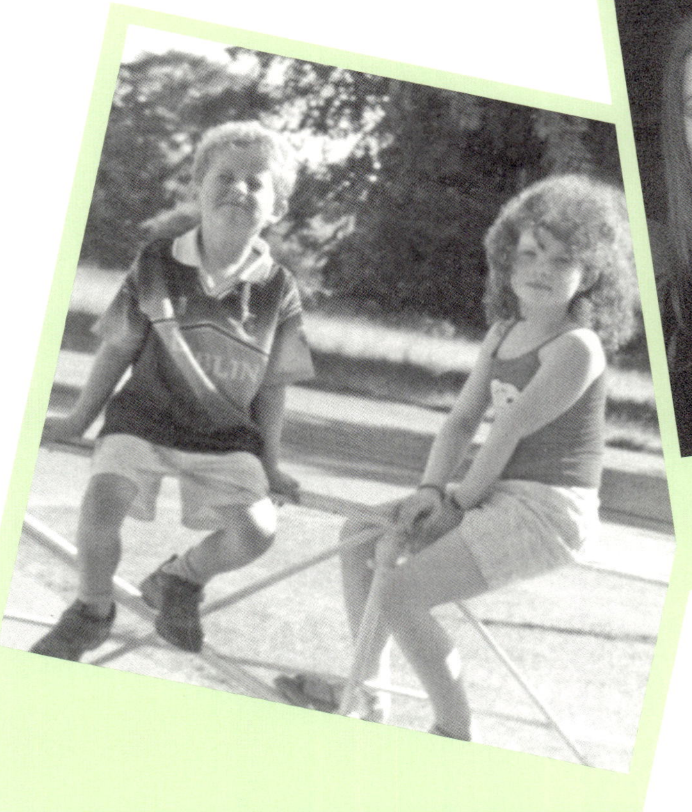

FIGURE 13: Final integration: A children's model of children's well-being

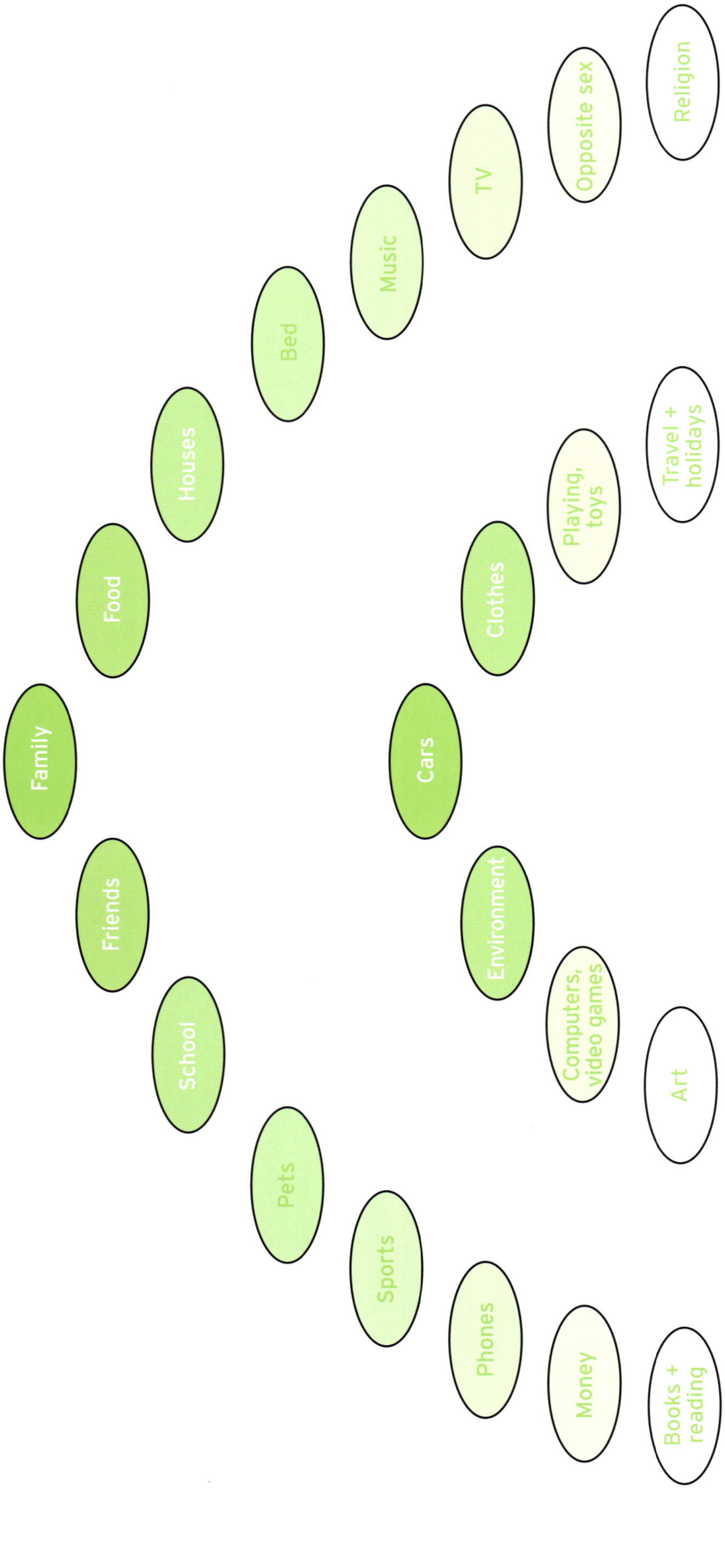

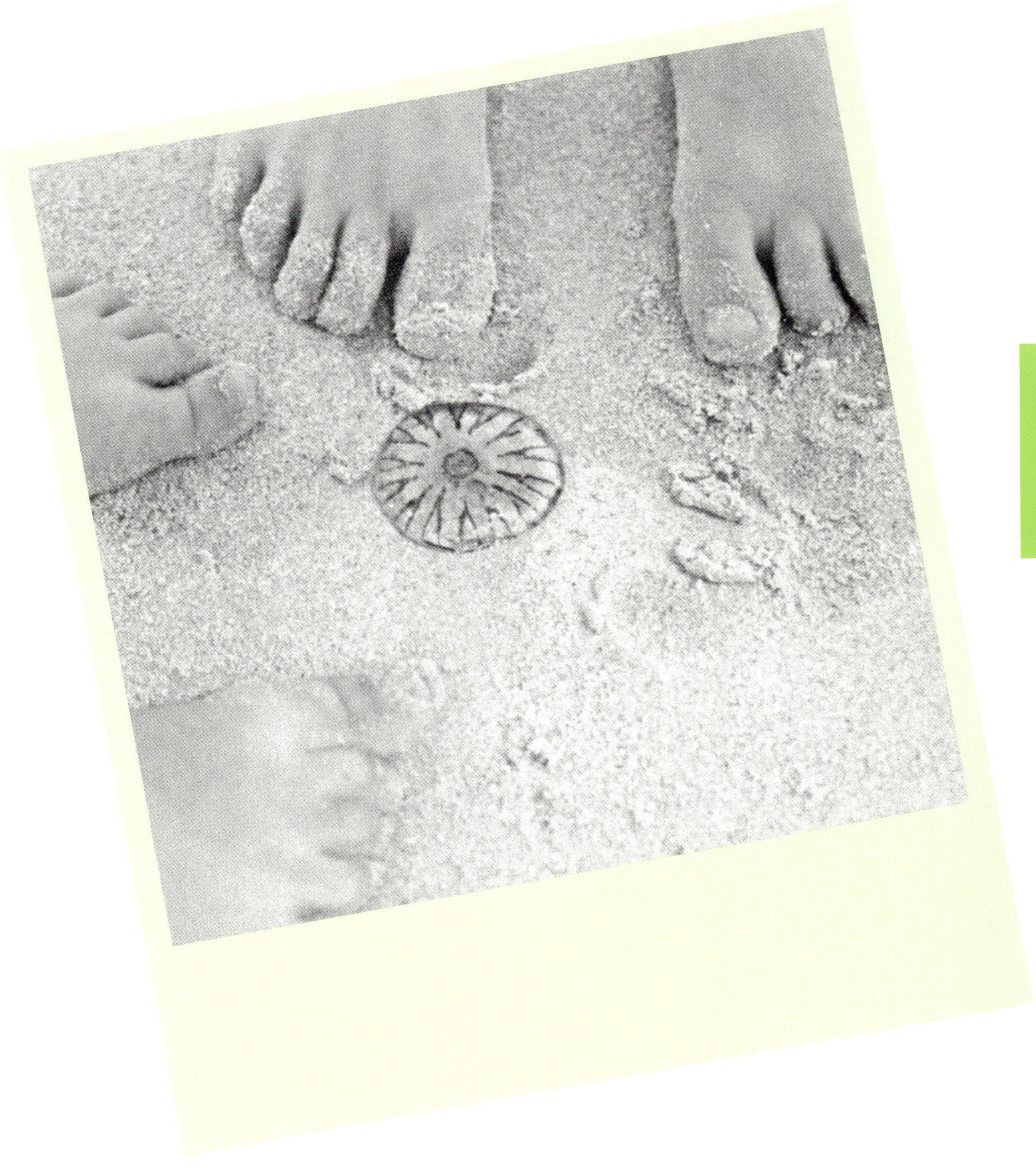

62

63

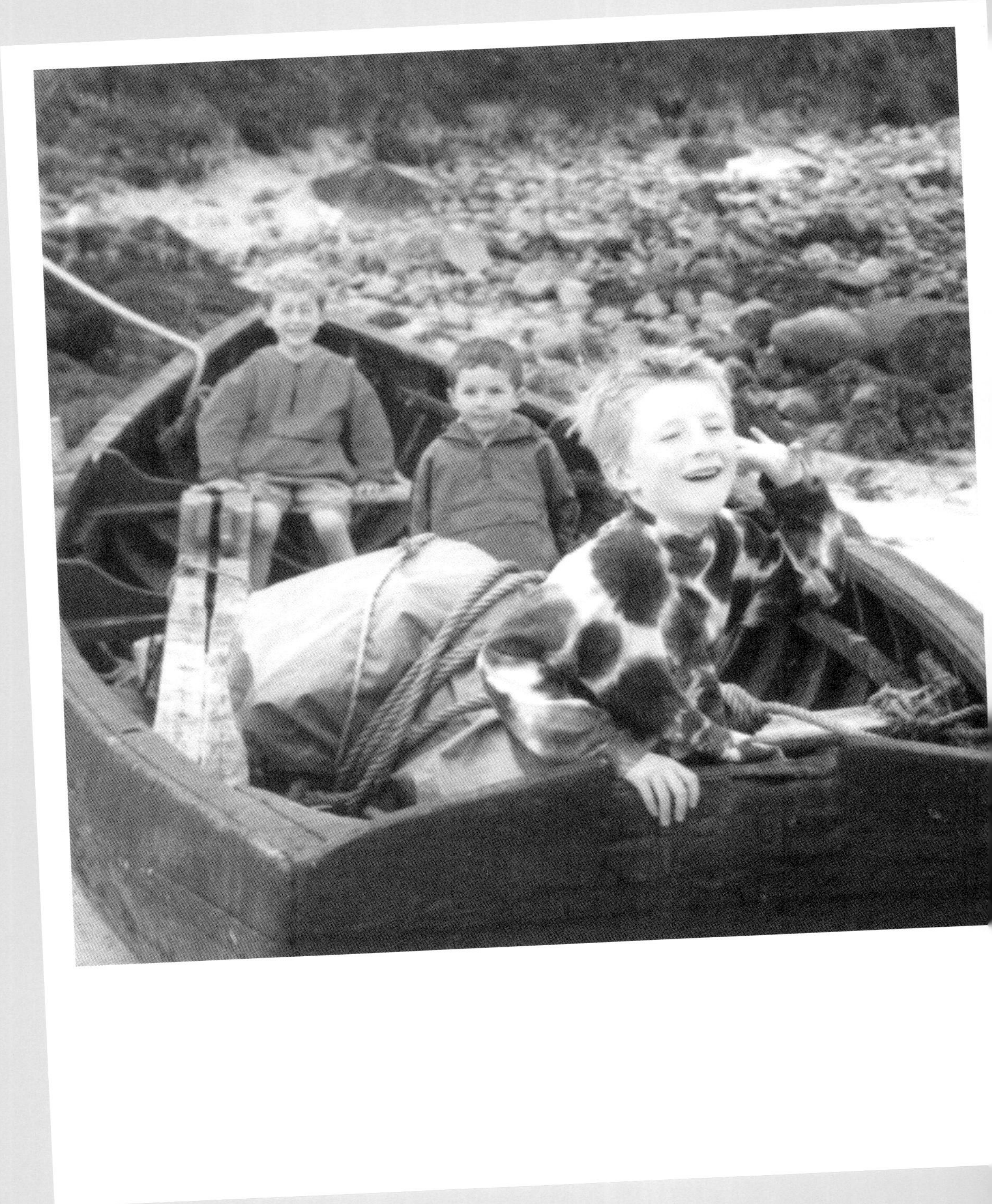

CONCLUSION

In this study, we have attempted to uncover children's understandings of well-being with the aim of contributing the perspective of children to the development of a national set of well-being indicators. To that end, the findings do illustrate most clearly the breadth of perspective that children have on this topic. The design and method of data collection is both novel and creative, and is therefore described in detail to support the credibility and confirmability of the findings. This study generated data of a very positive nature, both in terms of the subjects of the photographs and the discussion that they subsequently produced. In addition, and particularly during the schema development phases, the data illustrate the degree of complexity with which children understand the influences on their well-being to be interrelated. While in most groups, children developed hierarchical models without being prompted to do so and thus identified what they considered to be the most influential factors for their own well-being, they also spent considerable time in discussing and explaining the way they perceived the categories to be connected to one another.

A number of specifically interesting factors emerged during both the categorisation and schema development phases. The centrality of interpersonal relationships with family and friends (including school friends) emerges strongly, as does the value of activities or things to do. During all phases, children discussed how aspects of the various categories made them feel; how relationships (with people and animals) and the activities within or context of those relationships gave them a sense of belonging, being safe, loved, valued and being cared for. In a sense, this reflects a returning to the original explanation of well-being that was provided to those involved in taking the original photographs: *feeling good, being happy and able to live your life to the full.* While many of the categories identified may have been predicted from reviewing previous work and so validate these aspects, the categories of pets/animals and environment/places are relatively unexpected yet credible as they were confirmed by the different groups of children independently at the three stages of the study and integrated in the schema development when the opportunity was available to reduce their importance. These categories illustrate the extent to which children interact with the natural world around them, as well as the interpersonal environment in which they are located. These factors certainly deserve further attention from researchers, policy-makers and practitioners.

There can be no single 'true' understanding of a concept such as well-being, most particularly among children. Thus, in the plural 'understandings' we recognise the likelihood of multiple perspectives, which can be observed in the differences at the various stages of the process of data collection. Each phase represents an 'understanding' of well-being in its own right, as well as contributing to a final outcome – the integrated schema. It is likely that the developed schemata would be different if different children were involved in their construction. Nevertheless, it is of note that in both the second and third phases the same categories emerged across many groups *(see Table 4)*. Thus there is a certain level of robustness evident in the patterns emerging.

The differences that have emerged during each phase of this study between children from the various socio-demographic groups in some senses validate the approach taken. Differences in understanding as well as relevance of particular issues would be expected to vary by social and personal experience and the data presented here differ by gender and age as well as urban/rural environment. These groups were chosen based on earlier work with Irish children that indicated differences in well-being by gender and age but not social class (Glynn, 2002; O'Higgins, 2002; Kelleher et al., 2003). However, groups could have been constructed based on entirely different criteria, such as family structure, academic performance or health status.

The location of the final integration within the youth centre setting was deliberate. Older children were chosen with the expectation that they would bring a broader perspective to the process. In addition, the fact that the particular group had experienced group-building training was considered an advantage. The series of steps they were asked to engage in were complex and required their full engagement. There was some evidence from the data that members of this group did try to consider the views of other children as expressed in the schemata from phase 3 in their final integration. Nevertheless, they are a very specific group of youth and the outcome of phase 4 may have been very different if this had been undertaken by any other group of children or indeed professional researchers. As with other qualitative approaches, the findings should not be considered generalisable, but rather transferable to similar groups in similar settings. Thus it is important that the findings of this study are considered as a whole without undue reliance on the exact location of a category within the final integrated schema.

These findings have potential application in a variety of settings. They endorse the whole child perspective taken in the National Children's Strategy (2000) and the approaches being taken within the Social, Personal and Health Education (SPHE) curriculum, both at primary and post-primary level. They also point to appropriate issues that should be addressed, both at policy and practice level. While the importance of relationship building and maintenance skills cannot be overlooked, family support and infrastructural supports, for both schools and community development in its broadest sense, are also necessary if we are to maximise well-being among our children.

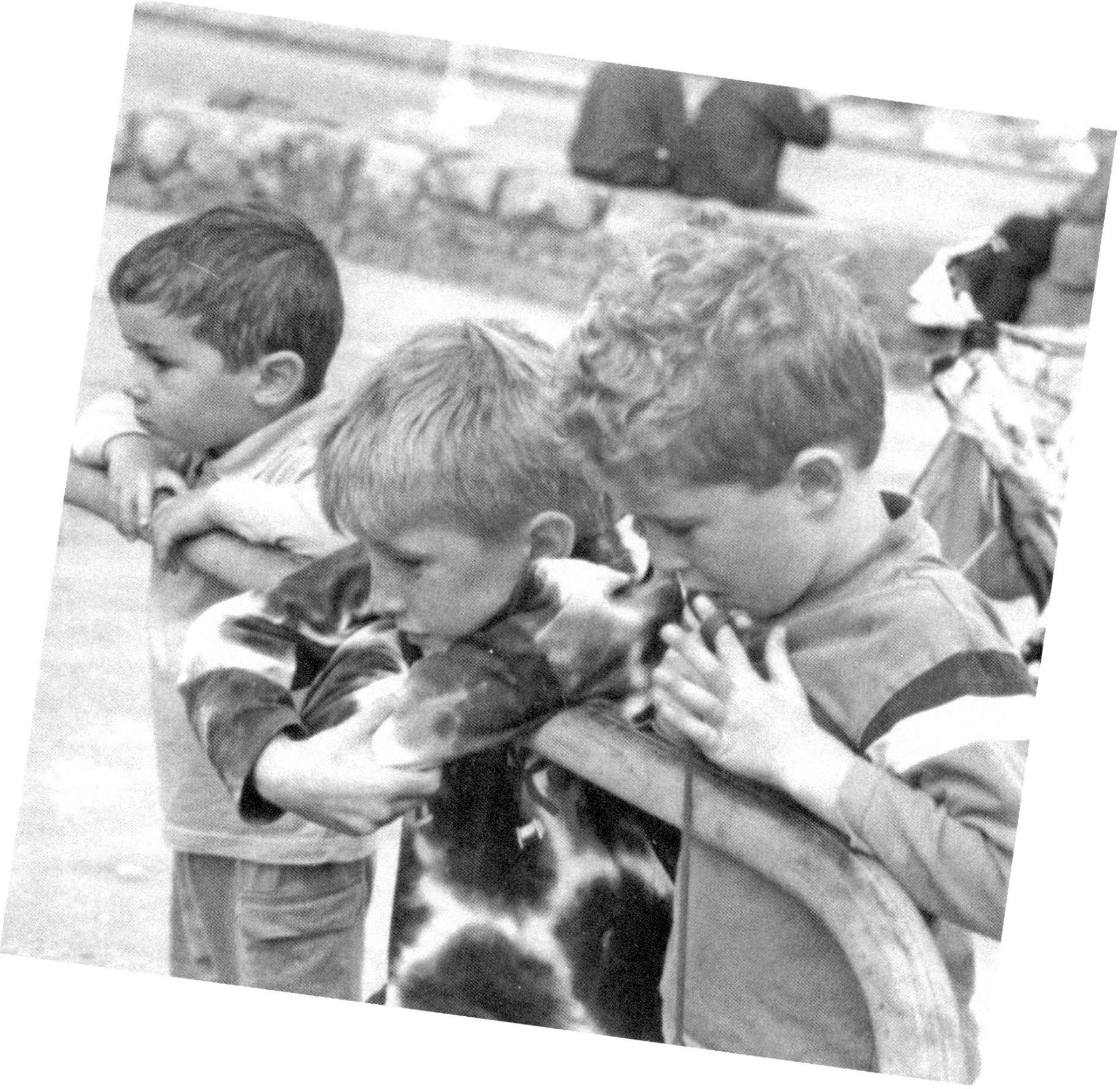

REFERENCES

Bowling, A. (1995) *Measuring Health*. Milton Keynes: Open University Press.

Diener, E. (1984) Subjective Well-Being. *Psychological Bulletin*, 95, 542-575.

Downie, R.S., Fyfe, C. and Tannahill, A. (1990) Health Promotion: Models and Values. Oxford: Oxford University Press.

Glynn, M. (2002) *Predictors of Positive Health in School-Aged Children*. MA thesis, Galway: Department of Health Promotion, National University of Ireland, Galway.

Huebner, E.S. (1991) Initial Development of the Student Life Satisfaction Scale. *School Psychology International*, 12, 231-240.

Kelleher, C., Nic Gabhainn, S., Friel, S., Corrigan, H., Nolan, G., Sixsmith, J., Walsh, O. and Cooke, M. (2003) *The National Health and Lifestyle Surveys: SLAN and HBSC*. Galway: Centre for Health Promotion Studies, National University of Ireland, Galway.

National Children's Office (2003) *A Study of Children's Understanding of Well-Being: Invitation to Tender*. Unpublished document, Dublin: National Children's Office.

National Children's Strategy (2000) *Our Children – Their Lives*. Dublin: The Stationery Office.

O'Higgins, S. (2002) *Through the Looking Glass: Young People's Perceptions of the Words Health and Happy*. MA thesis, Galway: Department of Health Promotion, National University of Ireland, Galway.

Tones, K. and Tilford, S. (2001) *Health Promotion: Effectiveness, Efficiency and Equity* (3rd Ed). Cheltenham: Nelson Thornes.

Torsheim, T., Samdal, O., Danielson, M., Dur, W., Hetland, J., Kostarova, L. and Valimaa, R. (2001) *'Positive Health'*. In Currie, C. (ed.) HBSC Protocol for the 2001/2 Survey. Edinburgh: University of Edinburgh.

United Nations (1989) *Convention on the Rights of the Child*. Geneva: United Nations.

Wilkinson, R.B. and Walford, W. (1998) The Measurement of Adolescent Psychological Health: One or Two Dimensions? *Journal of Youth and Adolescence*, 27, 443-455.

World Health Organisation (1946) *Constitution*. Geneva: World Health Organisation.